BEAUTIFUL
SKIN
BEGINS WITHIN

By Dr. Martin Braun, M.D. and Lorna R. Vanderhaeghe

Beautiful Skin Begins Within
Copyright © 2014 Lorna R. Vanderhaeghe, M.S.

Women Helping Women Communications
106A – 3430 Brighton Avenue
Burnaby, BC V5A 3H4

Library and Archives Canada Cataloguing in Publication
Vanderhaeghe, Lorna R.
Beautiful Skin Begins Within / Lorna R. Vanderhaeghe & Martin Braun
Includes bibliographical references and index.

ISBN: 978-0-9813517-7-3

The graph on page 43 is from Lorna Vanderhaeghe's *Healthy Fats for Life*, courtesy of Bioriginal Food & Science Corporation. All photographs on pages 79 and 80 are courtesy of Vancouver Laser & Skin Care Centre Inc.

NOTE: If you are taking prescription medications, consult your physician before applying the recommendations in this book. If you are on Coumadin of Warfarin, you should not change your diet, add any new drugs—either over-the-counter or prescription—or add any new supplements without consulting your physician.

DISCLAIMER: This publication contains the opinions and ideas of its authors and is designed to provide useful advice in regard to the subject matter covered. This publication is not intended to provide a basis for action in particular circumstances without consideration of a competent professional. The authors and publisher expressly disclaim any responsibility for any liability, loss, or risk, personal or otherwise, which is incurred as a consequence, directly or indirectly, of the use and application of any of the contents of this book.

COVER DESIGN: Barbara Burrows
INTERIOR TEXT DESIGN: Barbara Burrows
ILLUSTRATIONS: Katelynn Bailey
EDITORS: Krista Belli and Lisa Fukushima
ASSOCIATE EDITOR: Michelle Hancock
PRINTER: Friesens
Printed and bound in Canada
10 9 8 7 6 5 4 3 2 1
www.hormonehelp.com

ACKNOWLEDGEMENTS

From Lorna

Beautiful Skin Begins Within is my twelfth book and each
time I write a book I realize how many people are involved in
the process. This book would not have happened without my
coauthor Dr. Martin Braun, M.D. who has helped thousands
of women and men transform how they look and feel about
themselves. Our many discussions on the secrets to beautiful
skin are the foundation for this book. To my lover Trevor whose
support and encouragement always makes the process effortless.
To my family Kevin, Kyle, Caitlyn, Crystal, Max, Finn and Connor
and my six grandchildren; your love gives me strength.

To our editors Krista Belli, Michelle Hancock and
Lisa Fukushima, your attention to detail and thoughtful
comments ensure that this book will be easy-to-read
and full of interesting information. To our staff at both
Lorna Vanderhaeghe Health Solutions, Inc and the
Vancouver Laser and Skin Care Centre, you are all making
a difference in people's lives.

Contents

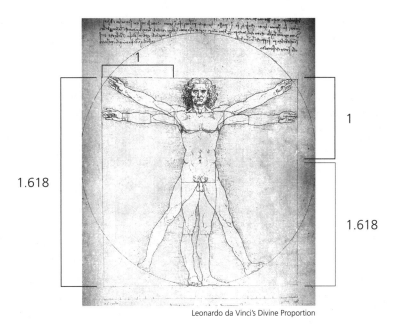

Leonardo da Vinci's Divine Proportion

The Golden Ratio of Beauty

While Dr. Braun and I were writing this book, he shared with me the mathematical equation behind the Golden Ratio of Beauty. It has long been said that beauty is in the eye of the beholder. But maybe our perception of physical beauty is hard wired into our brain and based on how our features meet the mathematical equations dating back to the days of ancient Greece. The ratio recognized as ideal is rounded to 1.6, and is called the Divine or Golden Ratio. It is known as phi in geometry, feng shui in Asia and Fibonacci numbers in India and this 1:1.6 ratio is nature's symmetry and occurs naturally in life in the way seed heads, pine cones, sunflowers and shells form and grow. Da Vinci used the Golden Ratio to draw the perfect body called the Vitruvian Man. The concept of the Golden Ratio is that the closer the object is to 1:1.6 the more beautiful we perceive it to be. A face or body with a ratio of anywhere from 1:1.5 to 1:1.7 is thought to be beautiful.

I found this interesting because I have a beautiful friend who has never been happy with her nose. After she had a rhinoplasty (a nose job) where her nose was designed to meet the Golden Ratio, she was so pleased with the way she looked. I have never liked my ears and have always worn my hair long to cover them. If the Golden Ratio is correct, maybe a simple surgery would change the way my brain views my ears. Dr. Stephen Marquardt studied human beauty in his maxillofacial and oral surgery practice. He developed the Marquart mask that uses phi and the Golden Ratio as the foundation for what we perceive as beautiful. He applied the rule to movie stars, models and people that we perceive as beautiful and over and over the mathematical ratios were clear in the distance between the length and width of the face, the center of the eyes to the bottom of the nose, and much more.

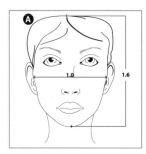

First measure the length and width of the face.
Then divide the length by the width. We perceive beauty when our face is about 1.5 to 1.7 times longer than it is wide.

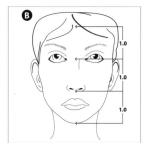

Next measure three segments of the face – from the forehead hairline to a spot between the eyes, from between the eyes to the bottom of the nose, and from the bottom of the nose to the bottom of the chin.
If the numbers are equal, a person is perceived more beautiful.

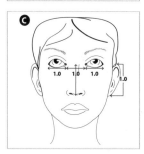

Other facial features can determine symmetry and proportion. On a perfectly symmetrical face the length of an ear is equal to the length the nose, and the width of an eye is equal to the distance between the eyes.

Dr. Lisa DeBruine of the University of Aberdeen Scotland found that female faces become more attractive to men when the women are ovulating. It may be that women might look healthier because they have a bit of a healthier glow when they are ovulating. Whatever our perception is of beauty, we know that smooth, glowing, radiant skin makes us feel more attractive.

It has been determined that we only have seven seconds to make an impression on someone when we first meet them. In those few seconds a person will evaluate your eyes, skin, posture and lips. If gorgeous looking skin, clear eyes and a beautiful smile can change the way we are viewed then we should go out and get it.

I teamed up with Dr. Martin Braun, M.D. because I love what he does in his clinic to help us look better and feel better. I first met Dr. Braun when my youngest was in her teen years. She was suffering with hyperhidrosis, also known as excessive sweating. It was a terrible problem that was affecting her self-esteem and social life. We tried all the natural and biofeedback options without success. I started researching what could be done to deal with the problem medically and after ruling out surgery to cut the nerves that send messages that cause sweating, I discovered that Dr. Braun was using Botox® as a medical treatment to stop the hyperhidrosis and it was covered by our medical plan. After one treatment she was free of the excessive sweating problem for 8 months and after a second treatment it never returned again. I also had a male colleague at the time who suffered from hyperhidrosis of the hands. As an executive, he was often in a situation to shake hands with someone but he couldn't because he was so embarrassed by the fact his hands were dripping wet. Dr. Braun also successfully treated his hyperhidrosis using Botox®.

Dr. Braun and I have teamed up in this book to provide you with the answers to your skin concerns. We know that if you take good care of your skin with nutrition, anti-aging nutrients and some of the skin smart topical agents we recommend, your skin will show less wear and tear as you age. And if you do decide to treat some of your skin conditions with cosmetic treatments, those treatments will last longer and you will get better results because you have optimized your skin integrity with better nutrition and lifestyle choices. The answers to taking ten years off your face are found in this book. No matter how old you are, you can have healthier, more beautiful looking skin. We guide you through the options available to turn back the clock—and there are many options. You will find everything you need to know about treatments that actually deliver results.

We have combed the research on nutrients that you can take orally or apply topically including vitamins A, C, E and coenzyme Q10 and plant extracts including sulforaphane as well as other botanicals. No skin book would be complete without discussing topical estriol, the only safe estrogen and one that has great research for smoothing wrinkles and halting unwanted male facial hair growth. You will never look at the ingredients in your cosmetics in the same manner. You will now be able to navigate the cosmetic department with confidence.

Dr. Braun's extensive experience in cosmetic rejuvenation is clear in the chapter on non-surgical cosmetic treatments. With lasers, natural fillers and methods to build collagen and elastin, we can have smoother and more youthful looking skin.

Our Beauty SOS chapter helps you understand your skin condition and how to successfully eliminate it. Whether it be the reduction of wrinkles, removing brown spots, eliminating cellulite, smoothing acne scars, removing unwanted hair, eliminating varicose veins, improving symmetry or building new collagen in the skin, this book provides you with smart solutions that work. Beautiful skin begins within the pages of this book.

CHAPTER 1: The Skin Within

Women with smooth, radiant skin aren't just lucky! They tend to follow the three secrets to beautiful skin. They nourish, protect and treat their skin. When you look in the mirror, you are actually looking at a mini-universe that is highly complex and sensitive to both internal factors like nutrition and hormones; and external forces in your environment including wind and sun. Your skin is your defender, your detoxifier, your temperature regulator, your insulation and your vitamin D producer. Let's *face* it: most of us don't care about any of this. What we want is smooth, flawless, glowing skin—and we are willing to do whatever it takes to have that beautiful skin.

The skin is the largest organ in the body and it is more than 30 layers deep and made up of numerous types of cells, each with their own important function. Your skin reflects your internal health. Dewy, smooth, blemish-free skin suggests that you are healthy, that you are drinking enough water, eating skin-supportive foods and otherwise leading a clean lifestyle that allows your body to work as it should to maintain hormone balance, to detoxify internally and to age gracefully.

Rashes, dry skin, acne, dark spots or puffiness are a sign the body is having health issues. Lifestyle plays a bigger role than genes when it comes to your skin, so if you are having skin problems ranging from acne to eczema or premature wrinkles, the good news is that we offer solutions that will improve the appearance of your skin and your overall health.

Our skin can also tell a lot about our age. *Can* is the key word because someone who follows a lifetime of skin smart habits is going to have younger looking skin than someone who does not. But thanks to billions of research dollars and the human desire and consequent efforts to "beat the clock," it is possible to stave off aging with topical, cosmetic and nutrition-based treatments that will leave people admiring and wondering, "Just how old are you?"

Be honest, you have already skipped ahead to the section in this book that applies to whatever flaw you perceive, or whatever beauty issue you are facing, haven't you? But first, it is important to understand the architecture of your skin so that when we later delve into particular interventions and treatments, you will understand *why* they work and what to expect if you choose these options for yourself. You will also be able to ask questions if you are working with a skin professional (and to answer questions when your friends ask what on earth you are doing for such fabulous skin). Understanding how your skin structure works is also essential to give you a firm knowledge base from which to judge marketing and advertising claims. The multi-billion dollar beauty business is all about selling products and services, and if you are going to spend money, spend it wisely, knowing that whatever product you purchase or treatment you choose is actually going to work. And don't worry we will make this quick.

Take the Skin Smart Test

First take our Skin Smart test. Be honest when you answer the questions. The answers will help you understand why your skin looks the way it does. You will need a magnifying mirror to get up close and personal with your skin.

My age _____

What your Mother can tell you about your skin
1.	My mother looks younger than her age	-1
2.	My mother looks her age	+0
3.	My mother looks older than her age	+1

What your Father can tell you about your skin
4.	My father looks younger than his age	-1
5.	My father looks his age	+0
6.	My father looks older than his age	+1

How you live can tell you about your skin
7.	I eat vegetables at least 3 times a week	+1
8.	I eat 2 or more servings of vegetables every day	+0

9. I eat 5 cups of vegetables every day   -1
10. I don't like vegetables and rarely eat them   +2
11. I eat fish twice a week   -2
12. I don't like fish or rarely eat fish   +2
13. I eat unsalted nuts and seeds 3 times a week   -1
14. I don't eat nuts and seeds   +1
15. I like fried food and eat it at least once a week   +2
16. I drink soda pop once or twice a week   +2
17. I eat soy foods   +1
18. I eat protein once a day (eggs, chicken, beef, protein powders)   -1
19. I eat protein two times a day   -1
20. I eat protein three times a day   -2
21. I drink at least 8 cups of water or herbal tea every day   -1
22. I don't drink much water   +2
23. I drink 3 cups of coffee per day or more   +2
24. I eat probiotic-rich yogurt every day   -1
25. I smoke   +2
26. I used to smoke but stopped more than ten years ago   -1
27. I like to tan in the summer   +1
28. I used to tan but no longer do so   +0
29. I go to tanning beds in the winter to keep up my tan   +2
30. I don't protect myself from the sun   +2
31. I protect myself from too much sun   -2

What does the mirror say?

32. The lines on the side of my eyes are only visible when I squint   -1
33. I have lines visible on the sides of my eyes even when I don't squint   +2
34. When I frown I get lines on my forehead but they disappear   -1
    immediately when I stop
35. I have lines on my forehead even when I am not frowning   +2
36. I have lines that only appear in between my eyebrows when I frown   -1
37. I have lines between my eyebrows that never go away   +2
38. I have lines that go from my nose to the corners of my mouth   +2
    (marionette lines)
39. I have a line under my bottom lip and between my chin   +2
40. I have lines above my upper lip   +2
41. When I lift the skin on the back of my hand it falls   -2
    back immediately

42. When I lift the skin on the back of my hand it slowly goes back in place   +1
43. My skin is red and/or has rashes   +1
44. My skin has brown spots or brown discolorations   +2
45. My skin is even toned   -2
46. The skin on my neck is moist and firm   -2
47. The skin on my neck and below my chin is looser than it used to be   +1
48. The skin on my neck is loose and sagging   +2

My Skin Smart Test Score: _____

If you have been skin smart, your score will be lower than 25.
If you are above 25, it is a good thing you are reading this book. The great news is we can reverse a lot of the damage done to the skin with diet, lifestyle changes and cosmetic treatments.

Under Your Skin

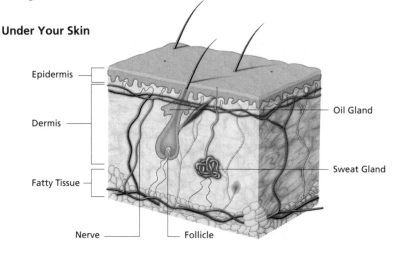

Epidermis

Dermis

Oil Gland

Fatty Tissue

Sweat Gland

Nerve   Follicle

The skin has three fundamental layers: the epidermis (the layer on top), the dermis (the middle layer) and the underlying fat layer (the bedrock). Within the epidermis alone are another four layers that help make this outermost barrier relatively tough.

The Protective Epidermis
Touch your skin and you are feeling the stratum corneum, which is comprised of almost 30 layers of dead keratin cells. Keratin is a protein also found in your hair and nails. These dead cells, or keratinocytes, overlap like

thick feathers on a duck and are interspersed with pores (ducts for sweat glands and hair follicles). Keratinocytes shed and regenerate on a never-ending basis. Old cells slough off and newer cells from below move to the surface at an average renewal rate of every 28 days. The younger you are, however, the faster your cellular regeneration rate generally is. This is why children and teens have that luminous glow that is indicative of swifter cell turnover. Once you hit your 20s and beyond, this process slows down and skin starts to look duller. But we can speed up cell turnover and you will learn how to do exactly that in the following chapters.

Changes in the way keratinocytes normally function accounts for the most common forms of skin cancer including basal cell and squamous cell carcinoma. Actinic keratosis is a pre-cancerous condition that shows up as red, dry, flaky patches in areas where excessive sun exposure has occurred. Skin cancers can be prevented by preventing sunburns. And thankfully, most skin cancers are easily treated when found early before they have spread to other areas of the body.

Skin Cell Turnover

BABIES AND CHILDREN: cells turnover every 14 days.

TEENS: cells turnover approximately every 21 to 28 days.

AGE 20 TO 40: cell turnover slows down to every 30 to 40 days.

AGE 50 AND OVER: cell turnover can slow to 1½ to 3 months.

Underneath the outer stratum corneum is a skin structure that resembles a stone-and-mortar wall. The "stones" are cells that will eventually shuffle upwards to the skin that you can see and the "mortar" is a mix of fatty ceramides (cell bundles) that are permeable to fats and oils, and love water and allow water-soluble molecules to enter them. Within this stone-and-mortar layer, the skin's soft keratin is made as opposed to the hard keratin of your hair and nails. Eventually this keratin will be sloughed away as dead skin cells.

Drop one level deeper into the skin and you will find a thin glue film that attaches the epidermis and dermis. In reality, the dermis is less than one millimeter beneath the skin's surface, yet it is this fingernail thickness that frustrates cosmetic researchers who are determined to sneak and slide active ingredients past this highly complex system of barriers, down to the dermis, where real change can take place. Yet the epidermis is crucial to skin integrity. A well-functioning epidermis is our best defense against harmful invaders like bacteria, viruses, foreign substances and toxins. It is also our protection against sun damage and possesses skin-plumping, anti-wrinkle properties.

The Dermis is the Difference

Finding ways to affect the skin's dermis is the focus of all skin care. The dermis is roughly twice as thick as the epidermis and is largely made up of collagen protein (a dense, foam-like filler) and elastin fibers that hold everything together in a way that allows the skin to flex and move. Collagen and elastin are what make skin plump and bounce back to the touch. When babies are born they are 90 percent collagen and this is why they have such beautiful, smooth, soft skin. Collagen and elastin float in a thick gel called hyaluronic acid. Hyaluronic acid is abundant in infant skin. Research has shown that hyaluronic acid is linked to reduced scarring and a reduction slows cell turnover. Hyaluronic acid levels in the skin increase in the presence of vitamin A (retinol) or retinoic acid (vitamin A acid); hence the reason why they should be used in skin rejuvenation.

Also found in the dermis are oil and sweat glands, hair follicles and nerve receptors, and blood vessels that carry nutrients and oxygen. In the following chapters you will learn how to build elastin and collagen and discover how fantastic hyaluronic acid, retinol and other skin nutrients are in improving the look and health of your skin.

When you look in the mirror and lament at large "pores," you are actually looking at either hair follicles or oil glands. Oil (sebaceous) glands are attached to hair follicles. Hair follicles are more concentrated in the T-zone of the face (across the forehead and down the nose) which is why the T-zone gets oily in some people. In the genital and underarm areas are the apocrine sweat glands. Also linked to hair follicles, these glands secrete sweat and body odor. Other sweat glands called eccrine glands are found all over the body and they help to regulate temperature. Botox®, a treatment used to smooth wrinkles, is used safely and effectively to halt hyperhidrosis or excessive sweating of these glands.

Like your epidermis, the dermis is constantly renewing collagen and elastin fibers and blood vessels. But as you age, and as exposure to the sun and environmental toxins damage the skin, this renewal rate can slow down. The hyaluronic acid cushion also diminishes. Touch a child's cheek and it is smooth and firm because they have ample collagen, elastin and blood vessels that supply cellular food and aid healing when the skin is injured. The untreated cheek of a 70-year-old will look and feel much different. Touch the cheeks of two 50-year-olds and they too will feel different, highlighting the fact that skin health—and health in general—is a very individual condition. Women in menopause are especially susceptible to collagen deficiency. Women lose as much as 30 percent of their skin collagen in the five years following menopause—and some women lose that much collagen in the first year after menstruation stops. And as if that is not bad enough, skin elasticity declines 0.55 percent per year after menopause. It is the loss of collagen that causes sagging skin and wrinkles. Fortunately, it is possible to support collagen production. In Chapter 4, we discuss the exciting research on beneficial nutrients that have been shown to enhance skin health and reduce the signs of aging. And in Chapter 5, we discuss laser treatments, dermal rolling and topical agents that help boost collagen and elastin production to stop wrinkles and sagging skin.

The Fatty Cushion Layer

Below the dermis, the third layer of your skin is the underlying fat layer. It is your skin's built-in shock absorber and insulates the body from cold. Pumping through this layer are larger nerves and blood vessels that feed the smaller ones in the overlying dermis. Large bands of collagen keep these fatty tissues in place.

Orange Peel Skin

Depending on the layout of that fat and collagen, the skin can take on a dimpled appearance. Dimpled skin is associated with the much dreaded cellulite. Cellulite can occur on any body shape, even in people who are lean and fit. We will discuss cellulite treatments in depth in Chapter 6.

Cellulite formation is caused by estrogen dominance and a poorly functioning lymphatic system. Blood is pumped through the body by the heart but your lymphatic system moves lymph and fluids by movement of the body. So those who sit are at a higher risk of developing cellulite.

A diet plentiful in skin smart foods, diligent sun care, appropriate beauty products and targeted anti-aging interventions can do a lot to turn back the clock. And as Dr. Braun often points out to his patients, the sooner you start with skin maintenance, the better. One of Dr. Braun's favorite stories is about a patient who is now nearing 40 but is constantly asked for identification at the liquor store. This patient has been taking care of her skin since her mid-20s and the effects of that early start are visible as she goes through middle age.

How Skin Protects, Renews and Repairs

Within the skin are several kinds of cells, each with a specific set of responsibilities. These specialized cells protect, renew and repair the skin.

▶ *Melanocytes* in the epidermis, hair follicles and retinas produce melanin, a pigment with the job of absorbing ultraviolet (UV) light from the sun. When you get a tan, what is actually happening on a cellular level is that UV rays have struck the skin and have triggered melanocytes to rapidly produce enough melanin to coat all the cells and protect them from DNA damage. A sunburn occurs when enough melanin cannot be produced quickly enough to stop damage to the blood vessels close to the skin's surface. Moles are a cluster of melanocytes that appear flat, round, oval or raised on the skin. We are probably all guilty of admiring a healthy-looking tan, but UV rays are a big contributor to premature skin damage and skin cancer, so practical skin sense is essential for long-term health and beauty.

Melanoma skin cancer develops when signals to the melanocytes become confused and mutation occurs. Sunburns not only increase aging but the risk of melanoma and other skin cancers as well.

▶ *Langerhans* cells are the skin's early warning system. Located in the epidermis and dermis, they alert the immune system and activate the immune army to destroy fungi, bacteria, or viruses or to protect an injury. When you cut your skin, Langerhans cells notify the immune system to send its army to destroy invaders and to heal the damage. The skin is the largest immune organ providing a covering much like plastic wrap protects food. Skin is tough and generally impermeable to bacteria and viruses. The skin also secretes antibacterial substances. These substances explain why you don't wake up in the morning with a layer of mold growing on your skin—most bacteria and spores that land on the skin die quickly.

▶ *Pluripotential* cells are found inside hair follicles. They are stem cells, meaning that they can develop into any other kind of cell—skin cell, collagen, immune cells—as needed. Once they become a specialized cell, they cannot transform again. Stem cell research is an exciting field of science that has the potential to reverse aging.

▶ *Fibroblast* cells are critical to skin health because they make collagen and elastin and therefore these cells are the most important components of skin structure. When your skin is damaged, fibroblast cells do the repair, replenishing collagen and forming scar tissue. As we age, these cells need more prodding to do their daily work; otherwise, they get lazy. When coveted collagen production declines, pits, rivers and valleys occur in the skin, which we call wrinkles.

FROM BIRTH TO THE GOLDEN YEARS: HOW DOES SKIN AGE?

What changes can you generally expect in your skin when you are 20, 40, 60, and beyond? These changes occur mostly in women who are not actively treating their skin from the inside out. The good news is we can prevent or treat most skin aging before it gets too severe—and if you think all that is left is a face lift, think again.

The Early Years: Soft as a Baby's Bottom

It is almost impossible not to want to touch a baby's soft skin. An infant's skin has a natural radiance about it because it is full of collagen, elastin and hyaluronic acid. And it is the hyaluronic acid that reduces scarring so that even if you cut your skin as a toddler you can rarely see the scars when you get older. Hyaluronic acid coupled with rapid skin cell turnover ensures children's skin is glowing and healthy looking.

Tumultuous Teen Skin

During puberty, flaring hormones contribute to acne and oily skin. Conventional approaches to teenage skin challenges include birth control pills and anti-acne drugs. Better options exist for those who want to get to the root of the problem and treat the underlying reason for acne instead of using a band aid approach. See page 83 for our recommendations for beating acne.

Twenties

If you were a sun worshipper in your teens, you may start to notice hints of sun damage—brown spots, broken capillaries and fine lines. You may also notice changes in your skin's luminosity. Your skin's cellular turnover rate is beginning to slow down. For some women acne does not abate in the twenties and becomes a chronic problem. It is important to rule out conditions, such as polycystic ovarian syndrome (PCOS), that are at the root of acne that continues in the twenties and thirties. But for most people the twenty-something years bring skin that is at its best.

Thirties to Fifties

You will probably notice some fine lines around the eyes and you may already have frown lines on your forehead. Your skin may be less lustrous. You may see brown spots on the sides of your face as these areas tend to get more sunlight. Hormone disruption, birth control use and an increase in progesterone during these years can exacerbate brown spots or melasma.

The shape of your face may also start to change, as fat decreases in the face, which can cause shrunken cheeks and less taut skin around your mouth and jaw line.

DNA damage in the skin now becomes apparent with pigment changes over larger areas. Brown spots, also called liver spots, appear on the back of the hands. Moles may darken. Spider veins appear on the cheeks, around the nose and the chin. Some notice varicose veins in the legs for the very first time in their thirties. Cellulite on the thighs and buttocks also becomes more noticeable.

Menopausal Skin

The average age of menopause is 52. Menopause means one year with no menstrual cycle. The decade leading up to menopause is called peri-menopause and the years following menopause are called post-menopause. Dramatic changes in the skin can occur at this time including sagging, wrinkling, increased pigmentation, acne, rashes, rosacea and more. During and after menopause, the skin clearly shows how wildly fluctuating hormones can affect skin tissues. Just like the teen years when hormones were raging, menopause creates challenges for the skin. Menopause can be viewed as a "multi-systemic" disorder of connective tissue. And connective tissue holds the layers of skin together. Low post-menopausal estrogen levels accelerate skin aging. High testosterone causes male facial hair growth. This affects both the epidermis and the dermis: fibroblasts not only decline, but they produce 30 percent less collagen. Estrogens act on collagen manufacture by directly stimulating fibroblasts. Topical estriol, the only truly safe estrogen, can prevent the post-menopausal loss of collagen—or eliminate it once it has started. All the solutions for menopausal skin problems are provided throughout this book so don't despair if you are already in menopause—and if you haven't got there yet, start a prevention program now.

Sixties and Beyond

During your 50s and into your 60s, most women notice increased blotchiness and redness, uneven skin tone and more broken blood vessels around the nose, cheeks and chin. Menopause can also dry out the skin which speeds the rate of collagen loss. We mentioned earlier that in the first five years after menopause, you will lose 30 percent of your collagen and some women will lose 100 percent in the first year, which will result in dramatic skin sagging and hollowness.

On the face and neck, you may observe increased sagging as collagen and fat redistributes in other areas. Above the eyes and under the chin, fat can accumulate. Women also tend to gain weight around the middle, the hips and on the buttocks.

Post-menopausal women may notice that their skin lacks luster and becomes dry, flat and dull looking. This is due to the inability to make gamma linolenic acid (GLA). GLA is a very special fatty acid that is the key to beautiful, glowing, soft skin. Before menopause the body can make GLA from the vegetables, nuts and seeds that we eat, but after menopause the enzyme that aids the body to make GLA no longer works and this is why our skin becomes dry, red, more prone to rashes and lacks luster. You will read more about this in the chapter on skin nutrients.

Your Skin As It Ages

AGE RANGE	MAIN SKIN CHARACTERISTICS
Early Years (infant, toddler, child)	Full of collagen, elastin and hyaluronic acid. Rapid cell turnover ensures beautiful, soft skin.
Teen Years	Hormone flare-ups contribute to oily skin and acne.
Twenties	The effects of sun damage become more apparent. Cellular turnover rate begins to slow down.
Thirties to Fifties	Fine lines and cellulite appear and the shape of your face begins to change. DNA damage is revealed through brown spots.
Menopause	Collagen production declines dramatically. Skin changes occur such as sagging, wrinkling, increased pigmentation, acne, rashes and rosacea.
Sixties and Beyond	Collagen content further declines and fat is redistributed to other areas. Women may notice sagging, red or blotchy skin and broken blood vessels around the nose, cheeks and chin.

CHAPTER 2: Skin Damaging

S kin is dynamic—it is constantly changing. There are no skin types in the sense that if you had oily skin as a teen, you will have oily skin as an adult. Or if you had dry skin as a child, you will have dry skin as you age. Or that you will always have combination skin. The state of your skin shifts constantly in response to numerous inner and outer factors such as your diet, your habits, your health, stress and your environment (we will discuss these shortly). Deliberately modify those factors and you can change your skin.

Sometimes, people are oblivious to the signs of skin in need. And remember, your skin is an indicator of your overall health. If you are constipated, your skin can become inflamed and develop rashes. If your liver is overwhelmed, your skin turnover will not be as effective and you can have more pronounced brown spots. Tune in to your skin (and the rest of your body) for the sake of your overall health and well-being. What is your current skin health? When you last looked at yourself in the mirror, perhaps you noticed persistent acne, an irregular breakout, or some other blemish that had you wondering, *what has triggered this*? If your skin was very dry, did you stop to ask why? Are you getting enough essential fatty acids? Are you exacerbating the problem with topicals that contain ingredients that may be doing more harm than good? Should you be using gentle products with anti-inflammatory herbs to combat skin flare-ups? Because skin is always in flux, yesterday's skin care routine may not be the best choice for today's skin. Follow our recommendations in the following chapters to ensure beautiful, glowing skin.

While skin is constantly changing—and may require changes in your habits and routines—it is possible to make generalizations about typical skin status. Very dry, dry, sensitive, normal, combination, and oily are classifications that you will commonly hear and see displayed on skin care products. These generalizations can be helpful because they provide clues about your health (and skin) status, as well as influencing factors. Certain medications, for instance, can be very drying to the skin. If you are suffering from chronically dry skin as a side effect of medication, a skin-supportive diet, nutritional supplements, and a high-quality moisturizer may help minimize the problem but not as effectively as avoiding the cause—in other words, improving your health and reducing your need for a prescription, or changing your prescription if necessary. Suppose your skin is rough and oily and prone to acne breakouts, especially during certain times of your menstrual cycle. This is often due to diet and/or underlying hormonal imbalances. Following a hormone-balancing diet will be an important part of your skin recovery, as will be applying appropriate topicals and developing habits that won't exacerbate the problem but, in fact, heal it.

UNDERSTANDING FITZPATRICK SKIN TYPES

Just as skin type generalizations exist (e.g. very dry to very oily) so do generalizations about common skin issues depending on your Fitzpatrick skin type, so named in the mid-1970s after Dr. Thomas B. Fitzpatrick. In dermatology, Fitzpatrick types are categorized by skin color, ranging from 1 to 6, and they describe how the skin reacts to the sun (ultraviolet radiation). These types can also reflect an ethnic connection. Do not confuse a tan with a Fitzpatrick type; you are born with the latter and it does not change throughout life.

Fitzpatrick Skin Types

TYPE	TONE	PIGMENT	SUNBURN
1	Pale	Pale white or freckled	Always
2	Light	White	Usually
3	Medium	White to Light Brown (golden)	Sometimes
4	Olive	Moderate Brown	Rarely
5	Brown	Dark Brown	Very Rarely
6	Black	Very Dark Brown to Black	Never

Of course, if you are a Type 1 or 2, you probably do not have to be told that you burn or develop freckles more easily than, say, your Type 5 friend, and you modify your sun habits accordingly. However, knowing your Fitzpatrick skin type can be beneficial because it provides clues about the skin issues more frequently affecting your type. Types 1, 2, and 3 are more prone to sunburn, redness, sensitivity, freckling and some hyperpigmentation (dark spots, or age spots). Type 4 is prone to general sensitivity. Types 5 and 6 are more prone to hyper-pigment or brown spots. Type 6 is also prone to hypopigmentation (skin lightening due to pigment loss) and keloids, which are excessive growths of scar tissue which can be flesh-colored, red or pink. The Fitzpatrick classifications have also given skin specialists a better understanding of how to use laser and light therapies. In the dermatologist's office, for instance, Type 1 and Type 6 patients will undergo different treatment approaches, as their skin types will respond differently to laser and light treatments for skin pigmentation and hair removal.

If you have not already taken our skin smart test to evaluate the health of your skin today, go back to page 2 and do so now.

- ▸ How does my skin look today? Is it smooth, beautiful, blemished, dry, saggy, wrinkled, stressed or irritated?
- ▸ Are there any specific areas of persistent concern? For example, blemishes, frown lines or a sagging chin.
- ▸ Have my lifestyle, diet, stress level or exercise patterns changed lately?
- ▸ Do I smoke or take medications?
- ▸ Do I have period problems?
- ▸ Am I in menopause?
- ▸ What kinds of skin and hair care products do I use, and do I use too many?
- ▸ Is my makeup the best kind for my skin?
- ▸ Do I touch my face too much? Do I pick at the acne on my face and/or back?

By identifying the influences that allow beauty to thrive, including the unique influences that specifically affect *your* skin, you can change what is not working or what is disrupting skin health, and take steps to achieve the smooth, glowing skin that you want in your retirement and beyond. So what are the most important factors that influence the skin?

FOODS THAT AFFECT YOUR SKIN
What You Eat and Drink

If you visited a dermatologist as little as ten years ago, you probably would have been informed that there was little or no connection between diet and skin health. Some still claim that there is a lack of scientific evidence on how the diet influences the skin. This kind of thinking has perpetuated the belief that you cannot do anything diet-wise for troubled, aging skin. This belief is far from accurate. Just as your diet can prevent cancer, ward off degenerative conditions, reverse diabetes and heart disease, and slow bone loss and aging in general, so too can your diet affect your skin.

A diet plentiful in dark colored vegetables and fruits, lean meats and fish, and essential fatty acids will benefit your figure, your organs and ultimately your complexion. Will one piece of wild salmon provide enough good fats to counteract a chronic skin condition? No. Will one basket of blueberries ward off aging, eye disease and inflammatory conditions? Unlikely. However, consistently supplying your body with the quality raw materials that it needs to perform as it should will reward you with smooth, radiant glowing skin—not to mention vibrant health and longevity. Eat too many junk foods, soda, alcoholic beverages, and refined, fried or processed foods or too few fresh fruits and vegetables, and you can expect to see premature aging skin and disease meeting your gaze in the mirror.

Your body is comprised of almost 100 billion cells, all of which are made up of proteins and fats. Carbohydrates are the fuel for these cells. If you do not eat enough protein—which is one of the main building blocks of keratin in skin—your skin will sag, your hair will fall out and wounds will be slow to heal. Or if you don't eat enough good fats, your skin will become dry and dull before its time, and your hair and nails will become brittle. Yet you need more than just fats, carbs and protein to survive and thrive. Other components known as micronutrients, including vitamins, minerals and plant nutrients, are also required for more than general health. In the skin, they help repair damage, build structures and maintain hydration. Although full-blown scurvy, which is a deficiency in vitamin C, is much rarer now than it was during the eras of long ocean voyages, most people do not consume enough of this essential vitamin. If you do not eat enough vitamin-C-containing foods like oranges, strawberries, lemons and tomatoes, or take dietary supplements containing vitamin C, your gums will become spongy, your hair follicles will bleed easily and you cannot make collagen. The effects of slow collagen production are visibly obvious when the skin loses its structure, sags and wrinkles.

Beyond vitamin C, many other nutrients play a role in how the skin functions (see a partial chart on page 17). Some good research has also been released on nutrition and skin health. One 2003 cross-sectional study looked at nutrient intake and skin status. The objective of the study was to determine whether nutrient concentrations were associated with skin health. Data was collected from 302 healthy men and women including the serum concentration of nutrients, dietary intake of nutrients, the hydration and sebum (oil) content and surface pH of the skin. The participants' skin condition was measured using non-invasive techniques, and their dietary intake was assessed using food questionnaires. After adjusting for sex, age and smoking, the researchers found that those individuals with higher levels of nutrients in the skin had better skin health. Higher serum vitamin A improved skin oil content and surface pH. A higher fat intake positively affected skin hydration and surface pH as well. In men, associations were found between the plant nutrient cryptoxanthin and improved skin hydration, and also between surface pH and fluid and calcium intakes.

SKIN NUTRIENT SUPERSTARS

NUTRIENT	ROLE
Vitamin A	A lack of vitamin A produces dry, scaly skin and increases the chance of infection. Vitamin A helps prevent acne, blemishes and possibly skin cancer.
Vitamin B	Required for new cell formation and protein synthesis; improves oxygen usage by skin cells.
Vitamin C	Prevents skin damage and anti-aging; required for the formation of collagen.
Essential fatty acids	Promote good skin elasticity and texture; required for protein production, cell growth and skin repair and improves moisture content (see pages 42 and 44 for more information on omega-3 and omega-6).
Iron	Required for oxygen transport to the cells, energy production and skin color. Low iron causes blue/black under-eye circles.
Selenium	Protects tissue elasticity; deficiency may lead to premature aging.
Zinc	Needed for wound repair, cell repair and for the production of genetic material and enzymes.

In another study in 2007, researchers looked at how nutrient intake could actually affect skin-age appearance. Using data from the first National Health and Nutrition Examination Study, they included information from 4,025 American women between the ages of 40 and 74. Nutrients were estimated from a 24-hour recall and clinical skin examinations were conducted by dermatologists. The women's skin was judged on wrinkling, dryness and skin thinning resulting in skin atrophy or sunken, sagging skin. It was found that women who consumed more vitamin C were more likely to have younger-looking, moister skin. A higher essential fatty acid intake was also associated with less dryness and skin thinning. Women who ate more processed carbohydrates and unhealthy fats, on the other hand, had more wrinkles and age-related skin thinning. These findings did not change according to age, race, education, sunlight exposure, income, menopausal status, body mass index, supplement use, physical activity or energy intake. The researchers concluded in *The American Journal of Clinical Nutrition* that healthy dietary behaviors benefit skin appearance and health.

Simply put, if you are told that what you consume does not affect your skin, this is outdated information. Just like every other organ in your body, the skin benefits from good nutrition. A whole-food, antioxidant-rich diet comprised particularly of those foods and nutrients in Chapter 3 supports beauty—and health in general—from the inside out.

Although we cover skin specific nutrients and formulas more in future chapters, it's important to mention here the necessity of a multivitamin/ mineral formula. We know that the standard North American diet does not provide adequate nutrients for optimal health. If you want to turn back the clock and/or improve whatever skin condition is troubling you, the first step is to fill in any nutritional gaps that are inhibiting your skin from reaching its smooth, glowing potential. You will need a foundational multivitamin/ mineral supplement in the most absorbable forms of nutrients available. A high-quality multinutrient formula like Multismart should contain vitamins, minerals, antioxidants and co-factors for enhanced absorption that:

- ▸ Neutralize free radicals responsible for premature aging
- ▸ Enhance cell turnover thereby preventing brown spots on the skin
- ▸ Encourage hormone balance
- ▸ Boost energy and endurance
- ▸ Balance blood sugar
- ▸ Promote proper digestion and nutrient absorption
- ▸ Enhance hair growth and thickness
- ▸ Encourage strong nails and bones

Your Hormones

Hormones are chemical messengers. They carry signals from one cell to another and regulate the function of their target cells. Hormones are supposed to be in balance. In an ideal world, this lock-and-key connective network flows effortlessly. More often than not, however, hormonal fluctuations cause skin upset. Remember the hormonal acne during your youth? At that point in life, the sex hormones—estrogen, progesterone and testosterone—are surging along with growth and development. Triggered by hormones to produce more oil, the sebaceous glands attached to hair follicles start raging. If hair follicles become clogged with dead skin debris, the oil has no way to be excreted and bacterial acne is the unfortunate result.

Hormonal acne, a concern of not only teens but perimenopausal women as well, occurs as a result of impaired ovulation during the menstrual cycle. Due to hormones in our food and environment, ovulation is disrupted and testosterone is abnormally secreted in excessive amounts causing acne around the hair and chin line, the chest and the back. This type of acne occurs around ovulation only to fade for a few days and reappear again. A common treatment for hormonal acne is the birth control pill due to its action of halting ovulation and impeding the secretion of testosterone. However, we do not advocate the birth control pill as a means of acne control. Many teenage girls go on the birth control pill when they are 15 and do not come off it until they are in their thirties. Today, one in six women of childbearing age are infertile and this epidemic of infertility may be attributed to years of being on the Pill. By combining nutritional supplements along with good skin care habits and targeted dermatological treatments if desired, acne can be reversed and the body can be supported nutritionally as well (see page 83).

Hormone flare-ups also occur during pregnancy and menopause. When a woman becomes pregnant, all those hormones naturally start shifting in anticipation of bringing a new life into the world. What follows for many women is nine months of unpredictable skin. Acne is possible due to the high levels of the hormone progesterone being secreted to keep a woman pregnant. As a result of the actions of estrogen and progesterone, some pregnant women also suffer from melasma, a brown discoloration above the upper lip and on the cheeks and forehead. Still other women report smooth, glowing reflections and lustrous hair, proving that every woman will have a different experience.

Although sweating and hot flashes are the top complaints during menopause, skin conditions can also flare up as a result of hormonal changes. A dull complexion can occur when lower levels of estrogen and progesterone result in less oil production and less growth of new blood vessels. Lower estrogen levels are associated with skin changes including dryness, reduced skin elasticity and collagen production, and skin thinning. Hormone replacement therapy (HRT) has been researched as a possible anti-aging treatment and, indeed, improvements in hydration, skin thickness and collagen levels have been observed. Estrogen also increases mucopolysaccharide and hyaluronic acid levels in the skin, which impacts skin hydration.

However, synthetic HRT is not the magic elixir of youth, nor do we advocate it for alleviating the symptoms of menopause. The famous Women's Health Initiative study revealed that the use of synthetic progestins and estrogens increased the risk of breast cancer, heart disease, stroke, blood clots and Alzheimer's dementia. Further research has shown that even short-term use can increase breast cancer risk immediately. And we cannot trust the bulk of studies that claim HRT is safe because these studies were not written by independent researchers but rather by writers hired by a drug company with vested interest.

Bioidentical, natural estriol is what we recommend topically particularly for wrinkled skin. Aging of the skin is associated with skin thinning, atrophy, dryness, wrinkling and delayed wound healing. These undesirable aging effects are exacerbated by declining estrogen levels in post-menopausal women. With increased interest in long-term post-menopausal skin management, studies on the restorative benefits that estrogen may have on aged skin have expanded. Estrogen restores skin thickness by increasing collagen manufacture while limiting the amount of collagen that is lost. Wrinkling is reduced following topical estrogen treatment since estrogen enhances the manufacture of elastic fibers, collagen type III and hyaluronic acid. Dryness is also alleviated through increased water-holding capacity, increased oil production and improved barrier function of the skin. Furthermore, estrogen controls local inflammation which is associated with skin wrinkling. Estrogen has also been found to accelerate wound healing, resulting in less scarring of the skin. For more information on estriol, see page 60.

Another hormonal factor linked to skin health is low thyroid function. Twenty-three percent of North Americans are currently taking thyroid medication and it is estimated that another 30 percent have yet to be diagnosed with low thyroid. Many people with low thyroid have not been diagnosed yet and suffer from common symptoms such as constipation, weight gain, cold hands and feet, and a thickening and yellowing of the skin. Eyebrows generally thin out, while hair on other parts of the body becomes coarse and brittle.

People with low thyroid also have brittle nails. Conversely, a hyperactive thyroid can cause a bronzed appearance and even melasma on the cheeks. Everyone should have a thyroid stimulating hormone (TSH) test every year. Your TSH should be between 0.5 IU/ml and 2.0 IU/ml. If you think you have an underlying thyroid condition read Lorna's book *A Smart Woman's Guide to Hormones* and visit www.hormonehelp.com for information on thyroid tests and natural treatments.

Genetics and Ethnic Background

Earlier we discussed Fitzpatrick skin typing as a way of getting to know your skin's strengths and weaknesses. Dermatologists also use this scale to help determine which laser or light treatments might be appropriate for a certain skin type or color. Still, while it's important to recognize this information, genetics and ethnic background do not guarantee how a laser treatment might affect your skin. If you have fair skin, you may be more likely to burn but, based on your lifestyle decisions (i.e. protecting yourself internally through an anti-oxidant-rich diet and supplements and externally through non-toxic sunscreen and sun-shielding clothing), burning is not inevitable. If your mother or father suffered adult acne, knowing what we know now about skin health, there's no reason why you are destined for the same fate. This book shows you how the best dermatological and nutritional treatments can prevent or prolong aging skin.

Health and Medications

Health radiates from the inside out. It's no coincidence that, when you have a cold or flu, your skin looks dull and your hair is listless. The body is putting the bulk of its energy into recuperation, relegating one's appearance to a lower level of importance. At the same time, the hair, skin and nails can be good indicators of what is going on internally. Athlete's foot, a fungal infection, can be an early symptom of diabetes, for example. When a disease or illness manifests externally and is recognized, it is an opportunity to address the underlying problem sooner rather than later.

If you are taking medication, your skin could be affected. Easy bruising is common in patients taking a daily aspirin or ibuprofen in order to lower their risk of heart attack. The birth control pill or excess progesterone can cause melasma or brown areas on the skin. It's important to be aware of the risks and manage any occurrences accordingly.

Sunshine and External Toxins

We have all had a sunburn at some time in our life, but some people are more susceptible to the sun's ultraviolet rays (UVA and UVB). UVB rays are the shorter of the skin-damaging rays and quickly burn the mid-layers of your skin. The damaged skin sends signals to the bottom layer of the epidermis, which responds by forming melanin to protect the active skin. It is the melanin that results in tanning and as the melanin remains higher in the skin you set up some natural defense against the sun but only after damage has been done.

> ### Lycopene Prevents Sun Damage
> Lycopene is a nutrient found predominantly in tomatoes and tomato-based products. In one recent trial, 20 women consumed 16 mg of lycopene daily for 12 weeks. After exposure to UV radiation, and in comparison to a control group, the lycopene group had significantly reduced skin reddening and inflammation.

Some skin experts would go so far as to recommend ultimate avoidance of sunshine. This recommendation is not as cut and dried as it was even five years ago. A little bit of sun can actually have a positive anti-inflammatory effect on skin conditions such as acne, psoriasis and eczema, where the immune system is inflamed. The sun's rays, ironically, cool the response of the Langerhans cells that direct the immune system. Our deep need of vitamin D, also known as the "sunshine vitamin," is another reason to enjoy a bit of sunshine. The body produces vitamin D when sunlight hits the skin.

Vitamin D is a critical nutrient for hormone health, cancer prevention and immunity, among other things. Many North Americans are low if not deficient in vitamin D. In spite of the sun's benefits, it is important to practice sensible sun care and to avoid a burn. With an estimated one in five people developing skin cancer during their lifetime, the days of slathering ourselves in baby oil and baking in the sun are long gone. We must balance our need for the sun's rays with common sense, erring on the side of prudence.

It is also essential to do everything you can to strengthen your body's immune defenses through diet and lifestyle, and to consume enough skin-protective essential fatty acids. Be aware of any suspicious skin changes (e.g. moles changing color, shape or size) and report them to your doctor. Avoid mid-day sunshine, wear skin-protective clothing when outside, and choose non-toxic topical sun care products that are rated by the Environmental Working Group, a non-profit organization in the U.S. that has judged more than 1,700 sunscreens, sunblocks, lip balms and moisturizers.

Their website at www.ewg.org/skindeep/ tells you what you need to know to find safe and effective sunscreens. "SPF" alone does not make a good sunscreen or sunblock. According to the EWG's latest analysis for their annual Sunscreen Guide, only one in five sun care products is recommended, compared to last year's one in 12. Their analysis considered factors such as what kind of protection the product offered (UVA, UVB or broad-spectrum), whether it was mineral- or chemical-based, whether SPF claims were overstated and whether risky additives were present. For treatments for sun damaged skin, read Chapter 5.

GLA: Our Internal Cosmetic
Although the skin always needs essential fatty acids, one study found that they are even more important during the summer after exposure to the sun. Experiments in Scandinavia found that GLA from borage oil significantly reduced UV damage to the skin. Participants in the study used 2,000 mg per day of borage oil. GLA is commonly used in skin care moisturizers to aid dryness, retain moisture of the skin and treat wrinkles. GLA is not found in fish or flaxseed oil. It is found in evening primrose, black currant and borage oil. Borage has the highest concentration of GLA at 24 percent. For more benefits of GLA, see page 39.

The skin being our protective layer against the outer world, it is exposed to a variety of other external forces such as wind and hot or cold weather conditions. These can have a drying effect on the epidermis. Were you to look at dry skin through a magnifying glass, it would resemble a hardened sponge. Staying hydrated internally and applying a topical moisturizer can help combat this problem. Essential fatty acids are crucial for internal protection.

Tobacco smoke is another airborne pollutant that prematurely ages the skin. It is often easy to spot a smoker by their rougher, duller skin and the wrinkled grooves around their lips. Among its other disastrous health effects, smoking causes the blood vessels to constrict, which prevents oxygen transport via the tiny vessels close to the skin's surface. Since cells need oxygen to survive, this causes cell death and slows cellular regeneration. Additionally, just like the sun, the toxins in cigarette smoke kill collagen and elastin. One Finnish study analyzed the skin of a group of smokers and lifelong non-smokers. The researchers found that non-smokers had a roughly 20 percent higher rate of collagen production and their cellular turnover rate was faster.

Stress and Sleep

Given the connection between stress and many diseases including cancer and cardiovascular disease, it will probably come as no surprise to hear that stress also impacts the skin. And when we say stress, what we really mean are the effects of a variety of stressors including trauma, pain, a difficult job, a family dispute, or even illness. If a group of ten people viewed the same stressful incident, their reactions would all be different. Those who reacted with extreme stress would undergo the most internal changes. Hormones such as cortisol and adrenaline would be pumping and the body would unconsciously be attempting to conserve energy for the heart and brain by drawing it from the extremities. While these built-in reactions are fabulous if it ever came time to outrun a tiger, for instance, they weaken the skin especially when the stressors are chronic and long-term.

Stress causes the heart rate, blood sugar and blood pressure to rise but unfortunately it suppresses immunity. Chronic stress has been shown to slow wound healing. In a 1995 study published in *The Lancet,* researchers found that caregivers who were responsible for caring for a sick relative were significantly (24 percent) slower at healing from a skin biopsy compared to a control group. Animal research has also suggested a link between chronic stress and a higher risk of developing skin cancer. Stress also exacerbates conditions like eczema and acne. When cortisol levels rise as a result of stress, the sebaceous glands are triggered to produce more oil. One study published in 2003 involving 22 Stanford University students found that those with the highest exam stress suffered the most acne flare-ups.

Yes, modern life is crazy busy and never seems to slow down, but good health in general—and skin health in particular—requires that we moderate our stress levels and adopt anti-stress strategies such as yoga, meditation, deep breathing or tai chi. Routine relaxation provides much-needed balance and actually slows aging at a cellular level due to its modulating influence on the immune response.

The importance of routine relaxation also explains why a good night's sleep is so valuable to health and beauty. When you sleep, your body takes a break, allowing your internal repair mechanisms to go to work. The sympathetic nervous system, which dominates when you are awake, rests while the parasympathetic nervous system kicks into gear, promoting circulation and oxygen flow. The skin benefits as repair begins, collagen is produced, and the toxins and fluids that contribute to puffiness (water retention) drain away. So what happens when you do not get enough quality sleep? According to the

National Institute of Health in the U.S., 40 percent of adults have sleep difficulties and women are more often affected than men. A lack of sleep compromises immunity, which contributes to premature aging. Without adequate rest, the skin also doesn't get a chance to heal and rejuvenate. A study in the *Journal of Investigative Dermatology* involving healthy women found that sleep deprivation disturbed their skin barrier function (i.e. how the stratum corneum prevents water loss and prevents foreign substances from penetrating). These stress-induced changes to the skin impacted inflammation factors known to play a role in psoriasis, eczema and atopic dermatitis.

Herbal Solutions for Sleep and Stress
If you have trouble sleeping, our recommendation is take a combination of melatonin (3 milligrams per day) at bedtime along with the herbs chamomile, hops, passionflower and valerian to promote a deep, restful sleep. Melatonin is a hormone manufactured from serotonin (our feel good hormone) and secreted by the pineal gland. Melatonin is also a potent antioxidant. The human body is governed by an internal clock that signals the release of many hormones that regulate various body functions. Melatonin is well known for its ability to control our sleep-wake cycles where it is secreted in darkness and suppressed by light. You must have a pitch black bedroom to secrete melatonin to aid sleep. Melatonin has been found to protect skin cells from the action of UVA and UVB rays. A 1998 study at the University of California also found that melatonin applied topically in combination with vitamins C and E reduced the damaging effects of ultraviolet light. Children have much higher melatonin levels than adults and, sadly, as we age it is dramatically reduced. Anti-aging specialists believe melatonin to be essential in retarding the aging process. Low levels of melatonin are also found in individuals with sleep and depressive disorders.

For insomnia sufferers, we recommend 5-HTP. 5-HTP is a precursor to serotonin, your happy hormone. Proteins in our food provide us with amino acids, one of which is tryptophan. Tryptophan is broken down into 5-HTP and then 5-HTP is turned into serotonin. A serotonin deficiency contributes to weight gain, anxiety, depression, sleeplessness and panic attacks. 5-HTP allows for natural sleep without the drugged feeling in the morning that can occur with prescription sedatives. 5-HTP has to be enteric-coated, which allows 5-HTP to be absorbed in the small intestine. If 5-HTP is not enteric-coated, nausea can occur when optimal doses are taken. Take a high-quality multivitamin/mineral supplement to ensure you get adequate levels of magnesium, vitamin B6 and vitamin B3 because these nutrients aid 5-HTP conversion into serotonin.

Summary

Your skin is influenced by a variety of internal and external factors, most of which you can control. Still other factors such as glycation and oxidative stress come into play and we will expand on them in the next chapter on nutrition. We hope it is equally clear that beauty starts from within and is a reflection of your efforts. If you are in your twenties, good for you for taking an interest in your skin before you are likely even noticing changes. If you see fine lines in the mirror, now is the time to take proactive measures, including eating more anti-aging foods, boosting your skin-supportive supplements, using skin products with ingredients that combat cell damage, practising sun sense and turning to dermatologic treatments if desired. The more effort you make, the better your results can be. We will discuss common beauty issues and integrated solutions in Chapter 6.

CHAPTER 3: The Glowing Skin Diet

Why accept aging when changing a few simple routines will shave a decade or more off your appearance, not to mention improve your health and ward off disease? Every year, when Lorna conducts her speaking tour across the country, she meets hundreds of women who have undergone startling changes as a result of adopting healthy choices. They have lost weight by reading *A Smart Woman's Guide to Weight Loss*. They have overcome PMS, abnormal PAP results, breast lumps, low thyroid, adrenal fatigue, menopausal complaints and many other hormone-related issues. Many women also look younger, year after year, which partly prompted the collaboration with Dr. Braun to write this book. These women are walking testimonials about the fact that it is possible to change your life—and consequently change your appearance. Happy, healthy and visibly glowing, these women had reclaimed their passion for life and, best of all, they were beaming with reclaimed self-confidence.

A smooth, luminous complexion starts with a diet rich in clean proteins, high-antioxidant fruits, good quality fats along with dark colored vegetables that are full of nutrients for our skin.

Milk May Not Do the Skin Good

A 2011 study by Nestle Nutrition Workshop Program found that milk and other insulin-promoting dairy products induced acne. Acne, which affects 85 percent of adolescents, can be regarded as an exaggeration of our insulin-disrupting diet. Milk products contribute to elevations of insulin-like growth factor-I, which then stimulates acne formation. Milk proteins are involved in increased male hormone production, clogging of the pores and blackheads, inflammation of the hair follicles and increased oil production. The researchers stated that restricting milk consumption would have an enormous impact on the prevention of diseases like obesity, type II diabetes, cancer, neurodegenerative diseases and acne.

Another study published in 2007 in the *Journal of the American Academy of Dermatology*, found when adolescent boys were put on a diet low in carbohydrates and processed foods they enjoyed a noticeable clearing of their acne. High glycemic index carbohydrates convert quickly to glucose (blood sugar), causing the body to produce insulin and male hormones (androgens), the latter of which stimulate oil production by the sebaceous glands.

Glycation and Oxidative Stress

Glycation refers to the process where glucose (sugars) attaches to the amino acids of tissue proteins in the body and produces new destructive molecules coined *advanced glycation end products* (AGEs). Ideally, in people with normal blood sugar levels, the pancreas produces enough insulin to push glucose into the cells and glycation does not occur. However, if blood sugar metabolism is impaired, AGEs can wreak havoc internally. AGEs have been shown to destroy the collagen in blood vessels (collagen is a structural protein found throughout the body not just in the skin), causing the vessels to harden thereby contributing to hardening of the arteries, blood vessel constriction and premature aging in diabetics. In the same way, AGEs have been shown to contribute to the breakdown of the skin's collagen, thereby reducing elasticity, increasing rigidity and the tendency to weaken which causes increased wrinkling. The acronym AGEs is a perfect description because this process ages us faster by causing brown spots, wrinkles and sagging skin.

HEALTHY BLOOD SUGAR CONTROL

For more than 25 years, a nutrient called Chirositol™ has been extensively studied at the Virginia Medical School. Over 30 published studies have been completed. Chirositol™, which contains around 95 percent D-chiro-inositol derived from carob, is a new nutrient for the treatment of insulin-resistant conditions including metabolic syndrome or Syndrome X, type 2 diabetes, polycystic ovarian syndrome, excess androgen-related conditions such as male facial hair growth in women, belly fat and weight gain. Chirositol™ is a molecule that acts just like insulin because it is structurally similar to insulin. By mimicking insulin activity, it helps control blood glucose levels, glucose storage and disposal of glucose in the cell. And it will not cause hypoglycemia or low blood sugar in those with normal blood sugar levels.

Chirositol™ has also been shown to reduce appetite and improve serotonin, our 'happy' hormone. Reduced serotonin or poor metabolism of serotonin is linked to increased sugar cravings. So by enhancing serotonin, Chirositol™ helps control appetite.

As if glycation was not bad enough on its own, the damaging effects of AGEs are connected to the increase in cellular waste and oxidative stress.

AGEs Speed Aging

Oxidative stress occurs both internally as a result of eating and creating waste, and externally on the skin. In the body, processes such as glycation produce *free radicals* that cause cellular damage and contribute to disease and premature aging. Externally, airborne pollutants and ultraviolet radiation are two common causes of free radicals that cause oxidative stress. In the skin, this can cause blotchy, red and brown pigmentation and can weaken skin structure which leads to sagging and wrinkles. Oxidative stress has been shown to break down collagen, alter cell renewal, damage DNA causing brown spots and mottled skin, and promote the release of inflammation factors that trigger inflammatory skin disease such as eczema, psoriasis, rosacea, dermatitis and rashes. Free radicals also contribute to the development of allergic reactions in the skin.

What is a free radical exactly? Think of rust for a minute. Slowly but surely, various chemical reactions occur and the result is an invasive corrosion that is the bane of every vehicle owner's existence! The damage created by free radicals in the body is like rust. Free radicals are a natural by-product of everyday reactions that produce energy for the body. Other major sources and generators include:

- Fried foods and heated oils
- Nitrates and nitrites in meats
- Toxic airborne chemicals
- Cigarette smoke, or smoke from forest fires
- Exposure to medical or electromagnetic radiation (i.e., computer terminals)
- Strenuous exercise
- Chlorinated water
- A high-fat diet
- Prolonged physical and/or emotional stress.

What these tiny molecules lack in size, they make up in destructive capacity. Many free radicals are highly toxic, mutagenic (cause cells to mutate) and carcinogenic (cause cancer). Stable molecules are held together by two electrons, but free radicals are missing one electron and thus they attempt to steal electrons from neighboring molecules. An undesirable ripple effect occurs in which more damage is created to other molecules in cells and cell membranes, and more free radicals are formed. Eventually, if left unattended, what was once comparable to a spot of rust becomes a car riddled with unsightly holes.

The good news is that it is possible to prevent harmful AGEs and free radicals from damaging the cells in the skin and throughout your body with powerful antioxidant nutrients and diet. Antioxidants are free radical scavengers. They readily disable free radicals, preventing healthy body tissues from being damaged. When the body is deficient in antioxidants, our risk of disease increases and aging accelerates. By eating foods rich in antioxidants such as vitamins A, C and E, selenium and phytochemicals (the pigments that give plants their colors), we can keep our defenses against free radicals strong and stave off their aging effects. A beautiful skin, anti-aging diet should be low in sugar but high in nutritional power, containing plenty of antioxidant disease-fighting nutrients. It's important to support the body with whole foods (preferably organic) that promote immunity and defend against cell damage. Focus on:

- ▸ Dark colored fruits and vegetables rich in vitamins, minerals and powerful plant nutrients known to fight cancer, heart and eye disease, and aging;
- ▸ Low-glycemic legumes (lentils, chickpeas) that metabolize into sugar slowly, thus protecting against the irregular sugar metabolism associated with aging, (pre)diabetic states, high cholesterol and hypertension;
- ▸ Root vegetables (garlic, onions) whose antioxidant properties fight free radical damage and help to lower blood pressure;
- ▸ Higher consumption of seafood and fish, which contain fatty acids that support cardiovascular health and prevent inflammation;
- ▸ Healthy fat choices, with olive oil being the primary food oil, and supplementing with GLA for further skin anti-aging benefits (see page 39);
- ▸ Lowered intake of commercially raised meat and dairy, which can spur inflammation;
- ▸ More fiber-rich fruits and vegetables that help stabilize blood sugar and support digestive health;
- ▸ Fewer processed, high-glycemic carbohydrates (e.g. white bread, white pasta, sweets and junk foods) that throw off blood sugar, cause weight gain, encourage insulin resistance and the development of AGEs;

▶ A good quality multivitamin/mineral formula containing essential vitamins, minerals, antioxidants and co-factors for added anti-aging protection.

SKIN SUPERSTARS

Be sure to incorporate the superstar foods in the following section into your diet. In the following chapter, we discuss the premier supplements to restore or keep your skin at its luminous, smooth and youthful-looking best.

Carbohydrates

Carbohydrates supply your body with energy. Your body converts all carbohydrates, with the exception of fiber, into glucose, a major source of fuel. Found predominantly in plant foods and, to a lesser extent, in milk and milk products, carbohydrates are divided into two groups: complex carbohydrates, which are made up of hundreds of sugar molecules linked together, and simple carbohydrates, which usually contain up to three sugar molecules.

Simple carbohydrates are usually identified by their sweet taste and are found in refined and processed foods. Simple carbohydrates include fructose (fruit sugar), sucrose (table sugar) and lactose (milk sugar). Although fruit is a simple carbohydrate, it is allowed in the diet in its whole, natural state. Fruit juices that no longer contain fiber are to be avoided (except for lemon and lime juice, which help slow the digestion of starches, thus lowering the glycemic index of foods).

Complex carbohydrates include fiber and starches, which are found in vegetables, legumes, beans, nuts, seeds and whole, unrefined grains. Fiber, found in plants, is another source of carbohydrates. Although you don't digest it, fiber is an important carbohydrate for sweeping the colon, thus preventing constipation; it also lowers blood sugar, cholesterol and triglycerides.

The worst form of carbohydrate is the refined type found in cookies, cakes, crackers and desserts. Refined carbohydrates offer empty calories and do not provide you with vitamins and minerals. Increase the number of complex carbohydrates you eat and reduce the refined carbohydrates. If everyone stopped eating white pasta, white rice, white flour and white sugar, diabetes, high blood pressure, high cholesterol and cancer rates would drop dramatically.

Within the complex carbohydrate category, there are foods that affect the rate of insulin release into the bloodstream. The glycemic index (GI) is a measure of how quickly carbohydrates raise blood glucose levels in comparison to a standard food (i.e. glucose or white bread). Too much insulin or too fast a release of insulin has health consequences and is linked to the development of diabetes, obesity and increased aging, so choose foods below 60 on the glycemic index.

Eat plenty of vegetables (good carbohydrates), especially the cruciferous vegetables: broccoli, Brussels sprouts, cauliflower, kale and cabbage. The nutrients in these vegetables help keep your liver healthy; they aid fat loss by detoxifying excess estrogens; and they provide bulk to eliminate constipation. Vegetables, most of which have a GI below 20, include non-starchy vegetables such as leafy greens, celery, broccoli, asparagus, avocado, tomatoes and sprouts.

Avocados and Healthy Fats

Healthy skin requires healthy fats, and avocado contains an abundance of the good fats that plump up your skin. Other sources of beneficial fats include fish, nuts, seeds and oils from plants including borage oil. Your skin requires moisture to stay smooth and even. Avocados also contain antioxidant nutrients including lutein, vitamin E, B-vitamins and potassium.

Vitamin E is the most important fat-soluble vitamin in the skin and it prevents free radical damage. Unfortunately, vitamins E and C are depleted when ultraviolet radiation from the sun damages the epidermis, which decreases the skin's overall antioxidant capacity and promotes aging. Eating avocados along with antioxidant-rich fruits and vegetables, however, can enhance the absorption of skin nutrients. A 2005 *Journal of Nutrition* study found that consuming avocados with carotene-rich foods enhances carotenoid absorption in the body. Even a small amount of avocado (30 g, which is just more than 2 Tbsp) added to a salad of carrots, lettuce and baby spinach, or to salsa, increased the body's ability to absorb skin-beneficial nutrients such as alpha-carotene, beta-carotene, lycopene and lutein.

Here are additional tips for ensuring you consume enough healthy fats:

- ▶ When shopping, choose coconut butter over lard and shortening.
- ▶ Skip all types of margarine.
- ▶ Choose healthy oils that are cold-pressed and organic.
- ▶ For low-heat sautéing, use olive oil, sesame oil or coconut butter.
- ▶ For salad dressings, use unrefined cold-pressed oils such as flaxseed, hemp seed, walnut, olive, sunflower, pumpkin seed or macadamia nut.
- ▶ For baking, use cold-pressed sunflower or safflower oil, butter or coconut butter.

▸ Don't fry foods. Frying promotes free radicals, which promote premature aging of the skin. If you burn the butter in a pan or cause oil to smoke, you have created cancer causing, skin damaging free radicals.

▸ Reduce your overall consumption of animal fats.

Berries for Beautiful Skin

The deep color of all berries is what provides their nutritional fortitude. Strawberries, raspberries, blueberries, blackberries, cranberries, açaí, goji—they all contain anthocyanidins, the red and blue pigments that provide color and belong to the flavonoid family. Flavonoids are anti-inflammatory, anti-cancer and antioxidant disease fighters. Flavonoids are able to alter gene expression in cells and repair DNA in the skin. Add a handful of berries to your morning smoothie containing protein powder, yogurt or water, and a banana.

Cranberries Are Great for the Skin and UTIs

In addition to being high in antioxidants, cranberries are an excellent treatment for urinary tract infections (UTIs). UTIs affect 80 percent of women at least once in their lifetime and they are a painful, often debilitating infection.

The proanthocyanidins, also called tannins, in cranberry inhibit bacteria from sticking to the bladder wall and halt the infection. Add one-half cup (125 mL) of unsweetened cranberry juice to a big bottle of water to make it more palatable.

Several studies found that whole cranberry provided relief for UTIs. Most cranberry products only use dehydrated juice which does not have the same benefit as whole cranberry containing the seeds, skin, pulp and lignans. A study in the *Canadian Journal of Urology* involved 150 women between 21 and 72 years of age who had recurring UTIs. These women were followed for one year and those who were given whole cranberry had a 44 percent lower incidence of UTIs than the group taking a placebo.

Look for whole cranberry combined with the probiotic *Bifidobacterium longum* (BB536) to help eliminate UTIs and reduce the need for antibiotic therapy with its side effects. BB536 has over 85 clinical studies and has been proven to prevent and treat Candida/yeast infections and to replenish good bacteria. BB536 has also been shown to reduce *E. coli*, the bacteria responsible for UTIs, and to prevent diarrhea and constipation. It is shelf stable so it does not require refrigeration and it is has the highest count of friendly, good bacteria found in these types of supplements. Probiotic Plus contains whole cranberry and BB536.

Vegetables That Bust Brown Spots

Brussels sprouts, cabbage, kale, broccoli, arugula, bok choy and cauliflower are all part of the cruciferous family. Cruciferous vegetables are unique because they provide high levels of powerful plant nutrients called glucosinolates, indoles and isothiocyanates which have been found to prevent and treat cancers and protect our DNA.

Penn State University researchers found that isothiocyanates may help increase sunscreen's ability to prevent deadly melanoma formation. Isothiocyanates, the antioxidant found in cruciferous vegetables, are inhibitors of a protein called Akt3 that plays a role in the development of 70 percent of melanomas (melanoma is a deadly form of skin cancer).

Scientists are very interested in the cancer-prevention and treatment potential for high intakes of cruciferous vegetables as well as the isolated indoles from those vegetables, especially indole-3-carbinol, diindolylmethane (DIM) and sulforaphane. Read more about indole-3-carbinol and sulforaphane in the next chapter. For now, do not forget to eat plenty of cruciferous vegetables for your skin and hormone health. Imbalanced hormones play a role in acne, rosacea, wrinkles, red and inflamed skin, brown spots and cellulite.

Super Antioxidant Green Tea

Both green and black teas are derived from the same plant Camellia sinensis. The manufacturing process is what makes them different. Green tea is produced by lightly steaming the fresh-cut leaf, so it is not fermented and green tea provides high levels of compounds called polyphenols that are known for their powerful antioxidant effect. Antioxidants prevent free radical damage to collagen, elastin and skin cells. The main active compound in green tea, epigallocatechin-3-gallate (EGCG) inhibits the inflammatory process—a process that damages the skin and can ultimately lead to wrinkles. Research has shown that green tea extracts help to reduce DNA damage to the skin. Drink organic green tea daily.

Lemons and Limes

Remember the skin is an extension of our digestive tract and poor digestion can lead to rashes, eczema, psoriasis and dull, dry skin. To get the digestive system working well, drink a cup of hot water containing some freshly squeezed lemon juice every morning before eating. Citrus fruits such as lemons, limes and grapefruits contain skin-supportive antioxidants including vitamin C, which is required for collagen production. Antioxidants prevent free radical damage and inflammation. Limonins, plant elements in citrus fruits, have been shown to fight skin cancer and other forms of cancer. According to the U.S. Department of Agriculture research, these compounds can stay in the blood for up to 24 hours whereas green tea compounds remain active for only four to six hours.

Moisturize Your Skin with Nuts and Seeds

It is worth repeating that essential fatty acids (EFAs) moisturize the skin, prevent aging, decrease wrinkles, treat acne and protect the skin from sunburn. EFAs are found in nuts and seeds and their oils; for example, flax seed oil, borage seed oil, sesame and extra virgin olive oil. Add unroasted, raw walnuts, almonds, hazel nuts, pistachios and Brazil nuts to your diet. Roasting nuts destroys their essential fat content.

People who consume more foods containing the good omega-3 fat alpha linolenic acid and vitamin C look younger in their later years, according to an *American Journal of Clinical Nutrition* study that examined the data of more than 4,000 women between the ages of 40 and 74. Conversely, if the women ate more processed carbohydrates and bad-fat foods, their skin was drier, appeared more wrinkled and was structurally weaker. These associations were independent of age, race, education, sunlight exposure, income, menopausal status, body mass index, supplement use, physical activity and energy intake.

Protein Stops Sagging Skin

Your body requires twenty essential amino acids to facilitate the production of protein for cellular repair, the manufacture of hormones, immune system factors, enzymes, and tissues. Of those twenty amino acids, twelve can be made within the body, and the remaining eight must be obtained from food. Two groups of proteins are found in your diet. Complete proteins—including meat, fish, poultry, cheese, eggs, milk, tofu, fermented soy and whey protein powder—contain all the essential amino acids. Incomplete proteins—including grains, legumes, and leafy green vegetables—do not contain all the essential amino acids.

Some people have greater protein requirements than others. If you are very active, exercise strenuously, do heavy labor, or if you are pregnant, you will need more protein than a couch potato. When choosing your protein sources, opt for free-range poultry and eggs, and wild fish over farm-grown fish, to avoid contamination from antibiotics and growth hormones. Purchase nuts in the shell and buy organic whenever you can. It is important not to choose toxic foods like bologna and hot dogs as your protein sources.

HOW MUCH PROTEIN DO YOU NEED?	
Adult men	70 g
Adult women	58 g
Pregnant women	65 g
Lactating women	75 g
Girls aged 13–18	62 g
Boys aged 13–15	75 g
Boys aged 16–18	85 g

The Benefit of Protein Powders

Protein is important for healthy skin. Consuming protein in the form of protein powders is an excellent way to get protein to help build collagen and elastin in the skin. Women who are protein deficient have sagging skin. If the skin on your upper arms is sagging, if your neck is heading to your chest or if your breasts are drooping, it may be that you do not eat enough protein. Women who sit in a chair and do no exercise require 30 grams of protein. An egg is a perfect protein and it contains 6 grams of protein. Knowing this, you can now see why most women are deficient in protein, which leads to sagging skin.

PROTEIN POWER SHAKE

1 cup plain, acidophilus, organic yogurt

1 scoop of your favorite protein powder

1-2 tsp GLA Skin Oil

½ cup fresh or frozen fruit, mango, papaya, berries or banana

1 cup water

3 ice cubes

Combine all ingredients in a blender, and blend until smooth. Drink immediately.

Powerful Pomegranate

Native to the Middle East and the Himalayas, pomegranate is a many-seeded fruit surrounded by a juicy, fleshy outer layer. The seeds possess anti-inflammatory properties by inhibiting enzymes responsible for inflammation and pain. As we learned earlier, free radical damage is one of the main causes of skin aging. Pomegranate juice has antioxidant power close to that of green tea and significantly greater than red wine. It contains an abundance of beneficial compounds including catechins, gallocatechins and anthocyanins. The most abundant polyphenols in pomegranate are called ellagitannins, which have powerful free radical scavenging properties. A food's antioxidant power is measured by its *oxygen radical absorbance capacity* or ORAC value. With a value of 105 ORAC units/gram, pomegranates beat out cranberries (93 ORAC units/gram), blueberries (77) and blackberries and raspberries (both 55).

Enjoy fresh pomegranates during the fall and winter, and look for the juice in the refrigerator section at your whole foods grocer. The juice has been shown to offer protection against cardiovascular disease and clinical gum disease. It also reduces the harmful products of lipid (fat) oxidation and reduces oxidative stress in diabetics. Although pomegranate juice contains sugars, in research with type 2 diabetics, pomegranate juice did not affect the patients' serum glucose levels.

Skin Calming Spices and Herbs

Nothing spices up a meal more than a few seasonings like mustard, cinnamon, chili, ginger, basil, sage, parsley, garlic, rosemary and thyme. And best of all, they are also great for skin. Most possess anti-inflammatory and/or antioxidant properties that fight free radical damage and premature aging to the cells.

Curcumin, the yellow pigment in turmeric, is a standout for skin care. Curcumin lowers the activity of cancer-causing agents while increasing their detoxification from the body. It is a potent antioxidant and anti-inflammatory agent. Due to its safety, efficacy and the variety of immune factors that it affects, it is also under consideration as a possible nutritional agent against arthritis, allergies, Alzheimer's disease and other inflammatory conditions. You can often find it in combination formulas for hormone balancing. Applied topically in a gel, curcumin can speed wound healing while reducing inflammation, redness, soreness and itchiness. Curcumin is being investigated as a treatment for various skin diseases like scleroderma, psoriasis and skin cancer.

Foods that Fight Inflammation

- Barley
- Beets
- Broccoli
- Cauliflower
- Cherries
- Cranberries
- Cucumber
- Grapes
- Hemp seeds
- Nectarines
- Olives
- Organic yogurt
- Pears
- Pomegranate
- Salmon
- Turkey

Foods for Glowing Skin

- Chia seeds
- Lemons
- Lima beans
- Limes
- Mackerel
- Mangosteen
- Oranges
- Organic chicken
- Oysters
- Peppermint
- Psyllium
- Pumpkin seeds
- Sardines
- Sesame seeds
- Strawberries
- Sweet potatoes

Foods that Boost Elastin Production

- Asparagus
- Black-eyed peas
- Brazil Nuts
- Celery
- Chickpeas
- Clams
- Dates
- Green peas
- Mangos
- Organic eggs
- Papaya
- Raisins
- Rhubarb
- Rosemary

Foods that Fight Wrinkles

- Açaí
- Acerola
- Almonds
- Apples
- Apricots
- Bell peppers
- Blackberries
- Blueberries
- Brussels sprouts
- Cantaloupe
- Carrots
- Green tea
- Flaxseeds
- Garlic
- Goji berries
- Kale
- Kiwi
- Onions
- Quinoa
- Spinach
- Sunflower seeds
- Tomatoes

CHAPTER 4: Skin-Loving Nutritional Supplements

You have just learned that food is the foundation for beautiful skin but can you get all the nutrients for beautiful skin from the food you eat? Or what if you want to reverse aging skin, enhance collagen production or increase cell turnover to get rid of those unwanted brown spots? This chapter highlights the researched-backed nutritional supplements that can reverse skin aging, boost cellular repair and create beautiful, glowing skin at any age. We have also included information on topical ingredients that have gained recognition for benefiting the skin. Along with a healthy diet, these supplements and topical agents can dramatically improve your appearance.

GLA for Glowing Skin
Essential fatty acids (EFAs) are the good fats that are essential for beautiful, dewy skin. Essential fatty acids are necessary for moisturizing the skin, preventing skin aging, decreasing wrinkles, treating acne and protecting the skin from sunburn. A deficiency in the fatty acid gamma linolenic acid (GLA) is the root cause of inflammatory skin conditions like dermatitis, psoriasis, rosacea and eczema. There is clear evidence that GLA has dramatic healing results when taken both orally and applied topically to treat all skin conditions from acne, cradle cap, wrinkles and itchy, scaling, dry skin. GLA contributes to the function of skin cell membranes where it helps to maintain the stability and fluidity of the natural water loss barrier in our skin to prevent substances from entering or irritating the skin.

GLA is found in borage oil (approximately 22 to 24 percent) and to a lesser extent in evening primrose oil (approximately 8 percent). The only human food to contain GLA is breast milk. After we are weaned, we make GLA from the food we eat. The earliest warning sign of a GLA deficiency is cradle cap in infants. Those people with eczema, psoriasis, dermatitis and dry skin are thought to have an impaired ability to make GLA from food. GLA is not found in food in high enough quantities to maintain our needs through diet alone and as such we should take a GLA supplement every day.

A recent study in the *Journal of Oleo Science* examined GLA's important moisturizing effect. GLA was given to adults with dry skin or mild atopic dermatitis and skin parameters were evaluated. The efficacy of GLA was demonstrated to be statistically significant in improving the skin barrier without side effects, and the researchers suggested that this is due to an anti-inflammatory action. In another study, patients given 500 mg of GLA per day for eczema had a 90 percent improvement over 12 weeks. Eczema is a common problem in infants and children. GLA is safe for all ages without the side effects seen with steroid creams.

Cradle cap and infant dermatitis or dry crusts occur on the scalp, face, armpits, chest and groin area and can be treated with topical GLA. In one study, 48 infants with dermatitis were given twice daily applications of GLA oil for six weeks with complete relief. One teaspoon containing 500 mg of GLA should be applied twice a day.

GLA has also been found to inhibit male hormones in the skin that cause acne. GLA can be taken both internally and applied externally to acne prone areas with excellent results.

In women who have gone through menopause, the enzyme that converts the food we eat into GLA becomes impaired and we can no longer make GLA. This is the reason post-menopausal women always have this dry, dull, lack luster looking skin. After menopause, it is essential that we take a daily dose of GLA to ensure beautiful skin. As we age, GLA can reduce inflammation in the skin associated with increased rashes, redness and dry, wrinkled skin. Without sufficient GLA, the skin becomes dry, rough and wrinkled.

GLA can be found in capsules and liquid form. Make sure the capsules you purchase have the actual amount of GLA in the capsule listed on the label. Most borage oil capsules tell you the amount of total oil in the capsule but are not so specific about the content of GLA. Ensure that the capsule does not contain soy oil either. Liquid forms of GLA are excellent because you get double the benefit; you can and should take GLA orally as well as apply GLA to the skin. GLA can be used in conjunction with your topical skin care products. Mix a little GLA into your favorite night cream or apply

GLA to the area under the eyes and around the mouth for maximum benefit. Lorna's GLA Skin Oil contains 500 mg of GLA per serving. The recommended dosage for individuals 90 pounds and above is 1 to 2 tsp (5 to 10 mL) daily and/or apply to the skin as needed. Always do a test spot on the skin when using GLA topically for the first time before you apply it everywhere.

GLA Challenge

For the fastest results, adults should take 2 tablespoons (30 mL) of GLA Skin Oil per day for 10 days and then reduce to the maintenance dose of 2 teaspoons per day. Your friends will be wondering what you had "done."

GLA for Skin Health

As a contributor to the healthy function of cellular membranes, the GLA found in borage oil helps to maintain the stability and fluidity of the natural water loss barrier in our skin to prevent toxic substances from entering or irritating the skin. Optimal structure and performance of the skin is necessary in order for it to function properly. When the barrier function of the skin is defective, skin disorders and damage can result.

Common skin disorders include dry skin, eczema, sunburn, acne and psoriasis. Dry skin is the most common skin condition and is characterized by rough, scaly skin and itching, particularly in the winter or in climates with low humidity. Dry skin is especially common in the elderly. By the age of 80 years, the epidermis may lose as much as 50% of its thickness, which accelerates water loss, leading to skin dryness. Dry skin also exacerbates many other conditions, including eczema and psoriasis.

Eczema

Atopic (allergic) dermatitis, or eczema, is a chronic inflammatory disease that affects up to 25% of the population and is characterized by dry, itchy and inflamed skin. The incidence of eczema has doubled in the last decade. Most people have dry skin to some degree, especially during winter and in climates with low humidity; however, those who suffer from eczema can experience itching so intense that they lose sleep at night, causing irritability and daytime fatigue. The itching, increased skin sensitivity and inflamed skin can induce severe skin trauma in which secondary infections can occur as a result of the scratching. See page 103 for SOS treatments for eczema.

Conventional Treatment for Eczema

Conventional treatment for eczema includes antihistamines, oral steroids, topical steroids and antibiotics to help control the symptoms of itching and inflammation. These drugs often have long-term side effects and are not recommended for continuous periods. A more natural and effective solution is needed to help provide eczema sufferers with the relief they so desperately need.

GLA: Keep Skin Moist

A dietary deficiency of the omega-6 linoleic acid (LA) results in a scaly skin disorder and excessive epidermal water loss. Because of the inability to convert LA into GLA (human skin lacks the D6D enzyme, which metabolizes EFAs), we become relatively deficient in healthy skin GLA.

Clinical research has found that people who suffer from eczema have low blood levels of GLA and increased levels of allergy-promoting inflammatory factors which may result in inflammation and itching. Therefore, supplementing with GLA is vital for keeping healthy skin cells moist and strong by improving the barrier function of the skin, reducing water loss through the skin, and acting as a powerful anti-inflammatory agent to reduce itching and inflammation.

Borage Oil: An Elixir for Eczema

Clinical trials have demonstrated that patients with eczema showed dramatic improvements with GLA supplementation. Andreassi and colleagues at the University of Italy set out to determine the effects of GLA from borage oil on the treatment of eczema in a study published in the 1997 *Journal of International Medical Research.*

Sixty patients with eczema (30 men and 30 women) participated in the 12-week trial. Of these, 30 patients were treated with 274 mg of GLA twice daily (one to two 1,000 mg borage softgels twice daily), while the remaining 30 received a placebo. Their symptoms were assessed by a dermatologist and by the subjects themselves every four weeks. Gradual and significant reductions in the itching, inflammation, blisters and oozing were noted in patients who received GLA in comparison to the control group. Some noted as much as a 90% improvement in symptoms following borage oil supplementation.

Patients receiving GLA were able to reduce their dosage of antihistamine and steroid therapies by 73%, antibiotics by 80% and the use of topical steroids by 50%. The investigators concluded that GLA supplementation in the form of borage oil is effective in the treatment of eczema, with noticeable benefits between six and twelve weeks. Borage oil does not produce the side effects common to antihistamines.

Borage Oil: Improves Efficacy
In another study, the effectiveness, safety and usefulness of borage oil on eczema was studied. Twenty-eight Japanese eczema patients were treated with 180 mg of borage oil daily for 4, 8, 12 and 16 weeks. The borage oil supplement reduced the symptoms of eczema with an increased effectiveness being noted with a longer period of treatment. Following 8 and 12 weeks of treatment, respectively, the researchers noted a reduction of 52.7% and 63.2% in symptoms, with a more significant degree of improvement being reported in the patients with the more pronounced symptoms such as itchiness, flaky skin and red rashes.

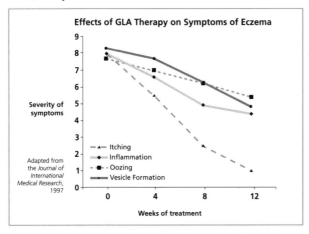

No significant side effects of the borage oil treatment were reported. The researchers concluded that their results indicated that borage oil appeared to be an effective and safe supplement, which could provide further control of eczema in combination with traditional medical treatments.

Borage Oil: Protects Mature Skin
Published in *Archives of Gerontology and Geriatrics* in 2002, researchers examined the effect of borage oil supplementation in 29 healthy elderly people with respect to skin barrier function, skin water content and fatty acid metabolism. Subjects received a daily dose of 360 or 720 mg of GLA (two or three 1,000 mg borage oil softgels) for two months. The barrier function of

the skin improved by an average of 10.8%, the water loss through the skin was reduced significantly, and the water content of the stratum corneum (outer most layer of the epidermis) increased slightly. Thirty-four percent of subjects suffered from itchy skin before supplementation, while no subjects experienced it after. The percentage of subjects who evaluated their skin as more dry decreased from 42% to 14% during the study. Increases of GLA and DGLA (the immediate derivative of GLA) from the borage oil were observed in cell membranes, with corresponding decreases of saturated, monounsaturated and omega-9 fatty acids.

The increase in the skin's water retention observed after borage oil supplementation may also counteract age-related decline of the skin barrier function and trauma due to scratching. As the study shows, borage oil counteracted itch in all subjects and itch is frequently observed in normal elderly people—even those without skin disease. Therefore, it is hypothesized that if supplementation with borage oil eliminates itch, scratching trauma would be eradicated, thus protecting the skin barrier function.

Recommended Dosage: Take one to two teaspoons of GLA Skin Oil or two capsules of GLA Borage Oil.

Calamari Oil Omega-3 Fights Skin Conditions

Calamari oil is very beneficial for many health conditions, especially where a deficiency in omega-3 fatty acids is a contributing factor to inflammatory conditions. Consumption of omega-3 fatty acids rich in EPA and DHA are known to decrease the inflammatory messengers in the skin and therefore they are invaluable in the treatment of inflammatory skin disorders such as eczema. Calamari oil is a sustainable, eco-friendly source of omega-3 fatty acids that comes from South American calamari (squid). Calamari oil is more stable than traditional fish oils, making it less prone to rancidity. Also, calamari oil does not cause fishy burps or unpleasant "repeating" that is common with fish oil supplements. Calamari oil is also higher in DHA, the fatty acid that is necessary for healthy eyes, heart and brain. DHA is the key fatty acid to stop dry eyes and it works wonderfully for dry skin as well. If you are concerned about impurities, PCBs, metals and other toxic substances in fish and fish oils but want the benefits of the omega-3 fatty acids then an excellent alternative is calamari oil. Calamari oil is much more ecologically sustainable because it comes from deep water, spawns quickly and multiplies fast. Because of their short life span, calamari does not have the same issues with mercury and heavy metal toxicity that fish do.

Recommended Dosage: To help treat eczema and dry skin, take two Cala-Q Plus softgels daily containing calamari oil with 720 mg of DHA and 50 mg of coenzyme Q10.

Psoriasis

According to the National Psoriasis Foundation, 7 million North Americans suffer from psoriasis. It is characterized by raised patches of red with white flakes or scales that appear on the torso, elbows, knees, legs, back, arms and scalp. When it is in the scalp, it can promote hair loss. In some, the nails may become dull, pitted or ridged and may separate from the nail bed. Psoriasis fluctuates between periods of inflammation and remission and is categorized as mild, moderate or severe. If the skin becomes too badly damaged, there can be fluid loss, bacterial infection and temperature dysregulation. Approximately 400 people die every year from psoriasis and another 400 are on disability pension. There are psychological ramifications as well, as people may feel shame, embarrassment, social rejection and anger due to a lack of understanding on the part of their peers. This psychological aspect can significantly affect relationships.

Psoriasis can also be associated with an autoimmune form of arthritis called psoriatic arthritis. There is pain, morning stiffness, swelling, reduced range of motion, pitting of the nails, tiredness and redness in the eye. In severe cases it can lead to deformity of the joints and spine. Difficult to diagnose in people with subtle symptoms, it is believed that 10 to 30% of those with psoriasis will also develop psoriatic arthritis. It usually appears between 30 and 50 years old.

Borage Oil: Sic it on Psoriasis

Most people find some relief with inflammation-reducing cortisone drugs, moisturizers and bath solutions; however, relief is only temporary. Psoriasis sufferers will be heartened to know that some publications and unpublished studies suggest that GLA may be effective in treating psoriasis.

For example, Dr. Darren Poncelet, a chiropractor and alternative medicine practitioner in Newmarket, Ontario, began using borage oil to treat patients with eczema and psoriasis as early as 1994. Since then, he has seen borage oil clear up almost all of the cases of eczema he has treated. He has also had some success with psoriasis patients, of which about 60% have found relief from their itchy, scaly symptoms. He has commented that some patients call it a miracle.

Dr. Poncelet has a nine-year-old patient with such an extreme case of psoriasis that she seldom went outside. When she did, she had to wear a toque, gloves and turtleneck to camouflage the weeping, bleeding wounds that covered her body. Her skin was raw and itchy and she shed two to three tablespoons of scaly flakes in bed each night. Poncelet prescribed borage oil softgel capsules. A year after she started treatment, his patient had noticed a "dramatic improvement." Her bleeding and weeping wounds had healed and the itching was cleared up. She is now able to enjoy the outdoors without having to worry about covering up; a year earlier that was only a dream. Poncelet says, "It's a huge emotional boost when they can wear shorts in the summer. She was elated the first time she went out."

Recommended Dosage: Take two tablespoons of GLA Skin Oil for 10 days and then reduce to the maintenance dose of two teaspoons per day.

Calamari Oil for Flaky Skin

Omega-3 fatty acids found in calamari oil and fish oil are potent anti-inflammatory agents that work to promote the remission of psoriasis symptoms. A study published in 2002 in the *Journal of the American College of Nutrition* confirmed that many trials of omega-3 fatty acids in chronic inflammatory diseases such as psoriasis and psoriatic arthritis reveal significant benefits, including decreased disease activity and a lowered use of anti-inflammatory drugs.

Recommended Dosage: Take 2 Cala-Q Plus softgels daily.

Cradle Cap

EFAs are critical for the healthy development of your infant. Up to 25% of infants may be affected with eczema later on in life. One factor suspected in the rise of allergies and eczema is a decrease in the number of breast-fed infants. Breast milk contains a blend of beneficial EFAs, especially GLA. Infants who are not breastfed may be missing out on this vital nutrient. In one study, the fatty acid composition of breast milk from 23 mothers of infants with eczema was compared to that of a control group with 18 mothers whose infants did not have eczema. The breast milk from mothers of children with eczema was higher in linoleic acid, but lower in GLA, DGLA and arachidonic acid compared to that of the control group. The researchers recommended doing further studies on GLA supplementation for breastfeeding mothers.

Infantile seborrhoeic dermatitis, or cradle cap, is described as dry crusts occurring on the scalp, face, armpits, chest and groin area, and it can be successfully treated with topical applications of borage oil. Research appearing in the *British Journal of Dermatology* in 1993 examined 48 infants with cradle cap who were treated twice daily with topical borage oil. The skin cleared up within 10 to 12 days, but lesions resurfaced within a week after treatment was discontinued. Treatment needs to be continued for at least 6 months. There were no relapses once treatment was stopped when the infants were 6 to 7 months of age.

This study demonstrated that borage oil is effectively absorbed through the skin and serves as a source of available GLA to reduce inflammation. Immature functioning of the D6D enzyme may be responsible for cradle cap in infants and can be corrected with topical or internal borage oil treatment.

In another study, when infants between one and seven months were treated with topical borage oil (0.5 ml oil per day) for cradle cap, they became completely free of all skin symptoms within three to four weeks. Conclusions were based on measuring the amount of water lost through the skin before and after treatment. The rate of water loss was restored to normal after the treatment. Improvements were even seen in areas where borage oil was not applied, proving its ability to penetrate and heal the skin as a whole.

Say Goodbye to Acne

Not only are teenagers challenged with peer pressure, hormonal changes, and life-altering decisions about college and careers, but approximately 85% of adolescents (20 million American teens) must also overcome acne. With heightened perceptions of their appearance and desires to fit in, teenagers can be emotionally and physically scarred by acne. In 30% of teenagers with acne, the acne will persist into adulthood. Acne vulgaris appears predominantly among teenagers and in women between the ages of 20 and 40 who cope with acne conglobata, a severe form of nodulocystic acne characterized by inflammatory lesions.

Acne is a condition that has affected most of us at some time in our life. It is caused by an increase in the production of androgens (male hormones) stimulating the oil glands beneath the skin to enlarge and increase the production of sebum (oil). Although they are male hormones, they exist in smaller quantities in women as well. The hair follicles, or pores in your skin, contain sebaceous glands (oil glands). These glands make sebum, the oil that lubricates your hair and skin. Most of the time the gland makes the proper amount of sebum, but sometimes the pores get clogged with excess sebum, causing the redness and eruptions seen as acne. Sebum moves along hair follicles to surface on the skin, and as it does, cells on the follicles are shed.

To prevent acne and maintain healthy skin, proper nutrition and circulation are vital. Healthy skin depends upon a consistent dietary intake of certain vitamins and minerals, as well as the right kinds of fatty acids. Deficiencies in essential fatty acids can cause an overproduction of sebum, resulting in acne. Research has shown that when the Inuit changed to the standard North American diet, they developed acne. Far less acne is seen in those eating traditional diets versus the standard North American diet, which is high in bad fat and refined carbohydrates like white rice, pasta and sugar. Eating too many of the wrong fats has also been shown to cause excess sebum production.

GLA and Acne: Help is on the Way!

Over 150 acne drugs exist: topical creams (such as Retin-A), antibacterial creams, antibiotics such as tetracycline, anti-inflammatory medications (corticosteroids), low dose birth control pills and Accutane. Some of these treatments come with serious side effects. Treating acne may be much simpler than taking hit-or-miss over-the-counter remedies, or harmful prescription drugs. In addition to eczema, psoriasis and cradle cap, natural treatments in the form of borage oil exist for acne as well.

Researchers explain that GLA from borage oil has the ability to inhibit androgens, male hormones that are present in men and women and are thought to cause acne, common baldness and seborrhea (skin lesions). GLA can reduce the symptoms related to acne, such as dryness, itching, oozing, inflammation and blister formation. Topically-applied GLA (from borage oil) in particular is showing great potential as a natural skin solution for androgen-related skin ailments. This statement takes into account symptom alleviation, as well as reduction in the use of prescription medications, including topical and oral steroids, antihistamines and antibiotics.

Recommended Dosage: Take two teaspoons of GLA Skin Oil or four capsules of GLA Borage Oil daily. Apply GLA Skin Oil to acne prone skin at bedtime.

GLA and Sunburn

You would be hard-pressed to find someone who has not had a sunburn at some time in their life, but some people (especially those with blond or red hair) are particularly susceptible to the sun's ultraviolet rays (UVA and UVB). UVB rays are the shorter of the skin damaging rays, penetrate deeply and quickly burn the mid-layers of your skin. The damaged skin sends signals to the bottom layer of the epidermis, which responds by forming melanin to protect the active skin. It is the melanin which results in "tanning," and as the melanin remains higher in the skin, you set up some natural defense against the sun but only after the damage has been done. A peeling burn occurs when active skin "commits suicide" and prematurely dies, creating extra top layers of skin which then peel.

UVA rays are longer, do not penetrate as deeply, but still cause damage. Often because sunblocks focus on absorbing UVB rays, you increase your exposure to UVA rays when you stay in the sun longer than you would without sunblock protection. The magnitude and total consequences of exposure to UVA rays is not fully understood, but it is generally agreed that UVA rays increase aging and wrinkling of the skin and perhaps more.

Sunburn symptoms will typically appear a few hours after overexposure—usually redness, swelling, tenderness and blisters. Following this appearance is a scaling of the outermost layer of skin. The symptoms usually peak within three days and their intensity will gradually diminish. The new skin, however, will remain very sensitive to sunlight for several weeks. The UVA and UVB rays induce a myriad of changes to the skin, including damage to the water loss barrier of the skin that results in loss of skin smoothness.

Although the skin always needs EFAs, they are particularly important in times of distress and damage, such as sunburn. Experiments on cultured skin cells show that ultraviolet light causes a significant release of fatty acids from cell membranes. The cell uses these fatty acids for the production of local hormones that regulate redness of the skin, swelling and pain. Typically, skin has a lot of arachidonic acid which, when released, exacerbates the severity of a sunburn.

When GLA from borage oil is given in the form of a supplement, it can quell the inflammatory effects of arachidonic acid. As a result, there is a reduction in the redness, swelling and pain that is created by the ultraviolet injury. Experiments on animals have proven that GLA from borage oil has the ability to restore the damaged water loss barrier, bringing back previously lost skin softness. In a Scandinavian arthritis study, 20 patients who received GLA from borage oil were also noticed as having significantly reduced UV damage to their skin.

GLA is normally taken orally and its concentration slowly accumulates in the skin. The process can be significantly accelerated if GLA is given topically as well as orally since GLA can be absorbed by the skin quite quickly.

Recommended Dosage: Take eight capsules of GLA Borage Oil or two tablespoons of GLA Skin Oil per day in two doses until symptoms subside. Borage oil can be applied topically to the skin two to three times daily.

Slow the Aging Process

Not surprisingly, GLA is also a skin beautifier for aging, dry and wrinkled skin. Through a variety of dietary and environmental factors and as the effectiveness of the D6D enzyme decreases with aging, it becomes more difficult for the body to produce GLA on its own. Without sufficient GLA, cellular membranes cannot lock in moisture and the skin takes on a dry and rough appearance. As we age or because of the various dietary and environmental metabolic roadblocks, we are at risk of losing GLA's moisturizing and anti-inflammatory benefits which produce a silky complexion and can soothe dry, scaly skin that may lead to wrinkles.

GLA is commonly used as an ingredient in skin care moisturizers and cosmetics to improve dryness, retain moisture of the skin, and help prevent the appearance of wrinkles. Ann Louise Gittleman, one of the premier nutritionists in the United States, and author of *Eat Fat, Lose Weight* and *The Fat Flush Plan*, recommends a GLA source from borage oil to all her clients to help them maintain healthy, glowing skin and prevent aging and wrinkles.

Recommended Dosage: Take two teaspoons of GLA Skin Oil or two capsules of GLA Borage Oil.

Other GLA Benefits

BONE DENSITY

Studies performed over 18 months found that when GLA was combined with calcium, it enhanced the absorption of calcium and improved bone density and prevented bone loss. Sixty-five women with an average age of 79 years were given 600 mg of calcium glycinate/aspartate along with 1,000 mg of GLA. These women had up to a 2 percent increase in bone density whereas the group receiving calcium alone lost 2 to 3 percent of bone density over the 18-month period.

BREAST CANCER

In a British study, women with advanced metastatic breast cancer taking Tamoxifen (a cancer drug that blocks estrogen) who also took GLA had a much faster response than those on Tamoxifen alone. Participants received 300 mg of GLA per day. The United Kingdom Cancer Research Campaign reports that GLA holds great potential in new cancer treatments.

CRAMPS AND BREAST PAIN

GLA deficiency is a major cause of PMS. A healthy body creates GLA via an enzyme from fats (such as sunfower oil) and in turn it is converted into prostaglandins, which are hormone-like compounds that regulate blood clotting, inflammation and muscle contraction. Just before menstruation, a cascade of prostaglandins are initiated in the uterus which causes the constriction of blood vessels and contractions that cause pain, cramps, nausea, vomiting, bloating and headaches that coincide with PMS. There are good prostaglandins and bad prostaglandins. Painful menstruation and breast pain are caused by low levels of good anti-inflammatory prostaglandins which are made from GLA. In many women with breast pain and terrible PMS, their ability to make GLA is often impaired. One trial done at the breast clinic at the University of Hong Kong used GLA for the treatment of cyclical breast pain. Of the 66 women in the study, 97 percent responded to treatment with GLA after six months. Further studies have found unusually low concentrations of GLA in women suffering with period cramps and breast pain. The recommended dose is 1,000 to 2,000 mg of GLA per day.

Collagen—The Foundation of Skin

The word collagen is derived from the Greek word "kola" meaning glue. Collagen is a structural component that makes your bones strong, your tendons elastic and your skin smooth. Collagen is the single most abundant protein in the human body. Proteins are made up of amino acids and collagen is no exception. When we are young collagen is produced in abundance and as we age collagen production declines. There are over 16 types of collagen, but 90 percent of the collagen in the body consists of types I, II, and III.

Collagen is essential to every structure in the body. When collagen production decreases, the muscles and skin sag, bones lose density, and the joints and ligaments become weaker and less elastic. Cartilage becomes thinner and weaker at the joints it is supposed to cushion. Hair loses its thickness and wave and breaks easily. Organs may sag toward the floor (prolapsed uterus and bladder) and sphincters weaken. The heart enlarges. Arteries become less elastic, more prone to aneurysm and become less resistant to plaque formation. Where we notice the loss of collagen the most is in the skin. Maintaining healthy collagen levels as we age will slow the structural decline of the body's tissues and organs.

Types of Collagen in the Body

Collagen is found in the majority of organs, not just the skin.

- Type I collagen—The most abundant collagen in the body. It is the strongest and toughest form found in tendons, bones, skin and other tissues. This type of collagen is abundant in scar tissue.
- Types II, IX, X, XI—Found in cartilage.
- Type III—Common in fast growing tissue, particularly at the early stages of wound repair which is later replaced with type I collagen.
- Type IV—Membrane of capillaries.
- Type V, VI—Generally found alongside type I.
- Type VII—Epithelial cells lining the GI tract, urinary tract and vaginal wall.
- Type VIII—Lining of blood vessels.

Stimulating New Collagen Growth

Skin rejuvenation treatments are designed to stimulate the development of new collagen. Lasers, intense pulsed light (IPL) and hyaluronic acid injections (which we discuss later) promote the growth of new collagen and there are also several research-backed nutrients that have been shown to dramatically increase the development of collagen in the skin as well.

Collagen in Nutritional Supplements

There are many different types of collagen supplements available: Type II collagen from chicken sternum and animal derived collagen from bovine or porcine sources; Type I, II, III and VII collagen from hydrolyzed marine collagen and elastin peptides; and gelatin from boiling the skin, tendons and ligaments of cows. Topical collagen agents are also being sold. So how do you know what type of collagen to use? Research has been performed using collagen for arthritis, wrinkles and bone health.

COLLAGEN CREAMS

The assumption behind collagen creams is that since the skin is made up of collagen, applying more collagen to the skin should increase collagen levels. Unfortunately collagen is such a complex and large molecule that it can not penetrate the skin. Building collagen from the inside out is the most effective way of enhancing collagen in the skin.

Collagen and Skin

Starting in our early 20s, collagen production declines by about one percent per year. Women in menopause are especially susceptible to collagen decline. Women lose as much as 30 percent of their skin collagen in the five years following menopause, which is the reason why we see bone loss, muscle decline, prolapsed uterus and bladder and skeletal aging in general. And as if that is not bad enough, skin elasticity declines 0.55 percent per year after menopause. The effects of slowed collagen production are visibly obvious when skin loses its structure, sags and wrinkles. A second yet equally important component of skin is called elastin. Elastin fibers form a matrix with collagen; together they allow the skin to flex and move. When we are young, the skin naturally renews its collagen and elastin. But with age and exposure to environmental toxins and sun damage, this renewal rate slows down.

Activated Collagen Reduces Deep Wrinkles in 28 Days

In a study of 43 women between the ages of 40 and 55 with crow's feet wrinkles, consumption of Active Collagen—containing types I, III and VII marine collagen and elastin polypeptides—was found to decrease lines and wrinkles and increase skin moisture. Two grams per day of either Active Collagen or a placebo were consumed for 84 days. The subjects' forearm and face skin conditions were measured at day 0, day 28 and day 84. Day 28 through 84 were during the winter months to simulate harsh winter conditions. After 28 days, the group taking Active Collagen showed a significant decrease in the depth of the number of deep wrinkles in 71 percent of the subjects. The placebo group, however, experienced an increase in the number of deep wrinkles at both day 28 and day 84. Active Collagen was found to have a powerful moisturizing effect on the skin whereas the placebo group had an increase in dryness. Active Collagen's effects just get better and better with women describing the crepe-like skin on their eyelids as smoother. The skin of the urinary tract and vaginal wall are made of collagen type VII, which is found in Active Collagen, so these tissues also improved.

The activated form of collagen used in the studies was sourced from European waters to meet the highest standards of purity, containing no shellfish or animal ingredients. Lorna's Active Collagen has the same ratio of collagen and elastin polypeptides present in healthy human skin. As you have learned, collagen and elastin are the two main components of the connective tissue in the skin. They have a synergistic, anti-wrinkle action: when taken orally, collagen and elastin stimulate the skin to lift and tone sagging areas and minimize lines and deep wrinkles. Health Canada has approved Active Collagen for reducing the number of deep wrinkles. It is rare for cosmetic products to be able to prove they can reduce deep wrinkles but Active Collagen can do just that.

Activated collagen can also increase the moisture level of dry skin and fight aging related to free radical damage. Marine polypeptides have a low molecular weight, making them water-soluble and easily absorbed by the cellular structure of the skin.

Vegetarians Can Enhance Collagen Too

The body needs the trace mineral silicon to make collagen. Silicon is converted into silicic acid in the digestive tract which the body then uses to manufacture collagen and elastin. Unfortunately, silicon from food, herbs and colloidal (gel) silica supplements is poorly absorbed, resulting in a lack of the building blocks required to make collagen. Silica gels are used to control moisture. You have most likely seen silica packs in bottles of drugs and supplements to keep moisture out of the bottle and never really given them much thought. Silica gel supplements do the same thing in the body, mopping up moisture and taking minerals along with it so we do not recommend silica gel supplements.

We know that, when ingested, silicon is converted to silicic acid, which is then used by the body to make collagen. But if you have poor digestion or if your body is not effective at converting silicon then you won't be able to make silicic acid and ultimately collagen. Impairment of collagen synthesis is a major contributor to excessive wrinkling in the skin. It would be much better if we could take silicic acid and that way collagen would be made directly from it. Thankfully silicic acid is available in nutritional supplements like Collagen Plus. Studies have been performed using silicic acid in women who had clear signs of sun-damaged or prematurely aging skin. In one study, women in the treatment group were given 10 drops of silicic acid daily for 60 days. Their skin showed significant improvement in wrinkling, improved elasticity and a significant reduction of brittleness in the hair and nails compared to the placebo group. Silicic acid is an oral cosmetic that should be used to enhance collagen production from the inside out. Collagen Plus should be used to prevent collagen decline in the skin and it should be used in conjunction with cosmetic treatments like IPL, lasers and hyaluronic acid fillers to increase and enhance collagen production.

Like silicic acid, biotin is important for healthy hair, skin, nails and bones.

Food sources of biotin include nuts, egg yolk, wheat bran, oat, barley, liver and brewer's yeast. However, the therapeutic amount of biotin required for healthy skin, hair and nails exceeds that found in the typical diet. Topical biotin, often added to hair care products, is not as effective as biotin in a nutritional supplement. Biotin has been found to increase nail thickness by 25% and reduce splitting. Collagen Plus contains both silicic acid and biotin in ideal doses for beautiful skin, hair and nails.

Pine Bark Improves Skin Elasticity and Hydration
French maritime pine bark extract is a potent antioxidant that fights free radicals. It has a high affinity for collagen and elastin, binding to them and protecting them from damage. In a double-blind, placebo-controlled clinical study with 62 women, a formula with pine bark as the lead active ingredient was shown to significantly increase skin elasticity by 9 percent after 6 weeks of oral treatment compared to a placebo. In addition, continuous intake of this formula for 12 weeks was shown to improve skin smoothness significantly by 6 percent compared to a placebo.

In a study published in *Skin Pharmacology and Physiology*, 20 healthy post-menopausal women supplemented with pine bark for 12 weeks. Before, during and after supplementation, their skin condition was assessed. Pine bark was found to significantly improve the hydration and the elasticity of skin. These effects were most pronounced in women with dry skin conditions prior to the start of supplementation. There was also a significant increase in an enzyme involved in hyaluronic acid synthesis as well as a noticeable increase in the pathway involved in collagen synthesis.

Improve Circulation in the Skin
Pine bark extract further improves micro-circulation to the skin by enhancing the body's production of nitric oxide, which causes the arteries to relax and consequently allows for optimal blood flow. Oral pine bark supplementation has been found to increase the delivery of blood and oxygen to the skin, resulting in improved wound healing in people with micro-circulatory disorders. Improved delivery of nutrients and oxygen supports better hydration and skin vitality.

Pine Bark Extract Protects Against Sun Damage
UV damage and photo-aging can be slowed by taking pine bark. Exposing the skin to UV light generates free radicals that in turn damage skin cells

and connective tissues. In an advanced stage, destructive processes cause an immune response which creates even more reactive cells that further degrade collagen and elastin. Pine bark, however, is anti-inflammatory and inhibits the trigger called NF-kB that governs the inflammatory response in immune cells. Oral supplementation with pine bark has been shown to inhibit the inflammation caused by UV-exposure and thus, it provides protection from sunburn.

Get Rid of Brown Spots and Hyperpigmentation

Other experiments suggest that pine bark helps to combat the problem of skin pigmentation. A clinical study demonstrated that pine bark is effective in lightening over-pigmented skin, also known as melasma or chloasma. Brownish spots or patches often develop on the female face, particularly in young mothers and in women taking contraceptives. Oxidative stress also contributes to this overproduction of skin pigment, and exposure to sunlight greatly contributes to further oxidative stress. However, supplementation with pine bark for one month in 30 women was found to significantly reduce the size of the area affected by over-pigmentation by 37 percent. Plus, average pigmentation intensity dropped by about 22 percent, proving pine bark is effective in supporting a fair skin complexion without side effects.

Studies have found that pine bark is effective for neutralizing a broad range of radical species. Pine bark also protects vitamin E from oxidation and recycles oxidized (spent) vitamin C back to its bioactive form, thus contributing to the antioxidant network in the body. After consuming pine bark for three weeks, the blood oxygen radical capacity (ORAC) of 25 volunteers increased significantly by 40 percent.

Sulforaphane Superstar Eliminates Hyperpigmentation

Eating cruciferous vegetables such as broccoli, cauliflower, kale and cabbage three to five times a week lowers the risk of cancer. What makes this vegetable group and the plant nutrients they provide so vital to skin health? Cruciferous vegetables provide indoles and isothiocyanates that maximize your skin cells' capacity to neutralize damaging free radicals and other toxins. In addition, one significant element called sulforaphane has been well researched for its ability to protect DNA in the skin and prevent cancer. Sulforaphane aids liver detoxification, which is important for detoxifying excess estrogens, environmental estrogens and other toxins from the body. Sulforaphane should be taken as a nutritional supplement because it is impossible to get enough from vegetables; you would have to eat 10 cups of raw broccoli per day to obtain enough.

Estrosmart for Every Woman Every Day

Sulforaphane along with indole-3-carbinol (I3C) should be taken by every woman every day. I3C is made in the gut when you chew and digest cruciferous vegetables. I3C is such a powerhouse that it helps break down cancer-causing estrogens into non-toxic forms and eliminates harmful environmental estrogens from the body. Like sulforaphane, I3C has been researched to prevent and treat cancer, and I3C has been shown to balance healthy estrogens in the body while supporting liver function. I3C also promotes a healthy cervix, protects against HPV cervical lesions and controls abnormal cell growth found in those with uterine fibroids and endometriosis. For the skin I3C halts hormonal acne, reduces inflammation and controls hyperpigmentation. I3C and sulforaphane are found in Estrosmart, a nutritional supplement we recommend every woman take every day, not only for hyperpigmentation but also for cellulite treatment and prevention.

Topical Sulforaphane Protects Against UV Damage

Sulforaphane can also be applied topically where it has been shown to repair damage, protect against future damage and reduce and soothe skin irritation. Its ability to stimulate detoxification and its antioxidant and anti-inflammatory properties all work together to prevent cell damage from the effects of oxidative stress and inflammation. In one study, sulforaphane-rich extracts from 3-day-old broccoli sprouts were applied topically to mice and human skin. This was found to repair UV damage through enhanced enzymatic detoxification, as well as to reduce UV-induced redness and fluid retention.

Topical Sulforaphane Counters Cancer Formation

Another study found that radiation-induced skin cancer formation was sub-stantially inhibited by extracts containing sulforaphane. After being exposed to UV radiation twice a week for 20 weeks, mice were treated with a topical broccoli sprout extract containing either low- or high-dose sulforaphane for five days per week for 11 weeks. At this time point, tumor incidence had reached 100 percent in the control group. The animal group that received the higher dose of sulforaphane had a 50 percent reduction in tumor burden, incidence and multiplicity. Tumor incidence and multiplicity did not differ between the low-dose treated group and the control group, but the low-dose sulforaphane treatment resulted in a substantial reduction of the overall tumor burden. The researchers concluded that topical sulforaphane-containing extracts are a promising strategy for protecting against skin tumor formation after exposure to UV radiation. Sulforaphane also accelerates the healing of sunburns when applied topically.

An interesting study looked at sulforaphane's impact on a rare skin condition called epidermolysis bullosa simplex in which the epidermis loses its integrity after mechanical trauma. Sulforphane was found to enhance the synthesis of the protein keratin, thus helping to restore skin integrity. Sulforaphane taken internally and applied topically on a daily basis will also reduce the pigmentation of brown spots on the skin.

TOPICAL TREATMENTS

The topical application of agents that offer both cosmetic and therapeutic benefit to the skin has been growing since the 1980s. Termed "cosmeceuticals," four general categories exist: exfoliating agents, whitening agents, antioxidants and regenerating products. We will discuss only a few of the most common ones here.

Alpha hydroxy acids promote shedding of the cells in the outer layers of the epidermis. The ingredients you will find in treatments and peels include glycolic acid, lactic acid, malic acid, tartaric acid, pyruvic acid and citric acid. They have all been shown to improve skin texture and reduce the signs of aging, as well as to treat sun damage.

Peptides are protein fragments created when collagen deteriorates in the skin. When peptides are identified by collagen-producing cells, these collagen producers order the body to increase collagen production to repair the skin damage. As you age, however, this mechanism breaks down, resulting in slowed collagen formation. The good news is, applying peptides directly to the skin has been shown to combat this problem and "trick" collagen-producing cells into producing more collagen.

As we have discussed, *hyaluronic acid* is a building block that fills out the space between collagen and elastin fibers in the skin, maintaining moisture and skin volume. Naturally, it is a popular ingredient for reducing the appearance of fine lines.

Antioxidants to Rescue the Skin

In the same way that dietary and supplemental antioxidants reduce and restore free radical damage and inflammation, so do they have the same protective effects on the epidermis when applied topically to the skin. Sulforphane and pine bark are just two nutrients that powerfully benefit skin health not only in supplement form but also when applied topically. Vitamins C and E, lipoic acid, coffee berry extract, coenzyme Q10, green tea extract, resveratrol, GLA, gotu kola, curcumin, pomegranate and marine-based ingredients are amongst the most commonly used nutrients in skin care products.

In one study, 20 women with photo-damaged skin applied a cream containing five percent vitamin C and 0.1 percent gotu kola daily for six months. By the end of the trial, they reported a significant improvement in skin moisture, softness, firmness and wrinkles.

A five percent vitamin C cream was tested against a placebo in another study involving 20 women between 55 and 60 years of age. After six months, dermatological and self-testing confirmed that their skin density improved, while the deep furrows on the sides of the neck smoothed out. It was concluded that topical vitamin C has a beneficial effect on aging skin. Topical vitamin C (at five percent potency) has also been found to reduce inflammation and redness caused by acne and rosacea.

Another trial involved the daily application of either a five percent alpha lipoic acid (ALA) cream or a placebo cream to 30 women with a mean age of 54 years. By the end of 12 weeks, the ALA group enjoyed not only visible skin improvements, but the researchers also used laser profilometry to test their skin and noted a 50 percent average drop in skin roughness compared to the placebo group. We suggest that you use a cream containing ALA and take 200 mg of ALA per day orally for optimal skin health.

Resveratrol is perhaps most well known for its heart benefits. However, topical resveratrol has been found to prevent skin cancer in mice exposed to a carcinogen.

Pomegranate extract is also found in anti-aging beauty products due to its antioxidant properties. The fruit contains an important plant chemical called ellagic acid, a powerful free radical scavenger. A 2003 study at the University of Wisconsin found that pomegranate extract inhibited skin tumors. Researchers looked at the application of pomegranate extract on mice against TPA, a cause of chemically induced skin cancer. The mice pretreated with topical pomegranate had substantially reduced tumor incidence and a lower tumor body burden. Thirty percent did not develop any tumors at all on the skin. Conversely, the mice not pretreated with pomegranate all developed tumors. Another 2010 study on the effects of pomegranate ellagic acid on both human skin cells and hairless mice found that pomegranate extract may protect the skin from wrinkles and inflammation due to sun damage.

Coenzyme Q10 Reverses Sun Damage

Coenzyme Q10, called the spark of life, is a well-known antioxidant nutritional supplement taken orally. But coenzyme Q10 has also been used in many skincare products for its anti-aging benefits. Research performed over ten years ago looked at how a lack of coenzyme Q10 affected aging skin and damage from chronic UVA and UVB sun exposure. Researchers at the Paul Gerson Unna Skin Research Center in Hamburg, Germany discovered that by increasing coenzyme Q10 in the skin, they were able to prevent sun damage. Coenzyme Q10 was also found to effectively penetrate the layers of the epidermis and reduce the depth of wrinkles. Coenzyme Q10 was also found to protect the skin against UVA sun damage.

Until recently it was unknown how and why coenzyme Q10 was so effective when applied topically to aging skin. Research published in the *International Journal of Cosmetic Science* in 2012 discovered that topical coenzyme Q10 increased collagen type IV production as well as elastin development, making skin smooth and firm. Interestingly, coenzyme Q10 also reduced the melanin content in the skin which has the potential to offer de-pigmentation effects for brown spots, melasma or sun damaged skin.

Coenzyme Q10 and vitamin A or Retin-A when used together have been shown to further reduce the damage produced by sun exposure and aging. Coenzyme Q10 applied topically along with your Retin-A cream should be part of your daily skin care regimen.

Estriol for Wrinkles and Male Facial Hair Growth

Estriol (E3) is a form of estrogen and it is the only safe estrogen. Unlike other forms of estrogen such as estrone and estradiol, estriol will not cause breast cell changes nor will it thicken the uterine lining. This bioidentical natural estrogen helps those women who are suffering from menopausal symptoms, especially urinary incontinence, thinning of the vaginal wall and vaginal dryness. Estriol can also be applied topically to the face to reduce the amount of male hormones in the skin, such as testosterone, thereby diminishing male facial hair growth. As you have learned, estrogen deficiency may be a common and important factor in skin aging. Estriol has also been found to improve the skin's density and turn old-looking skin young again by increasing the luminosity that gives us that youthful glow.

Estriol is so safe and effective that it is even used in wrinkle creams in Europe. In one study investigating the use of topical estrogen on the skin, 59 women with skin-aging symptoms applied a cream containing 0.3% estriol. Estradiol, follicle-stimulating hormone and prolactin levels were measured monthly along with skin hydration. In 10 patients, skin biopsies were taken to examine collagen levels. After six months of treatment, elasticity and firmness in the skin had markedly improved and wrinkle depth and pore size had decreased by 61 to 100 percent in both groups. Furthermore, skin moisture increased and the measurement of wrinkles revealed significant, or even highly significant, decreases in the depth of wrinkles in the estriol group. Collagen fibers also increased. As for the body's hormone levels, only prolactin increased significantly and no systemic hormonal side effects were noted.

Another study had similar findings and demonstrated that topical estriol is superior to estradiol for improving female skin aging symptoms. Eight patients were treated with a 0.3% estriol cream and 10 patients used a 0.01% estradiol cream for six months. Dermatologic follow-up was performed monthly. At each follow-up, prolactin (PRL), follicle stimulating hormone (FSH) and estradiol levels were sampled. In addition, prior to and after three and six months of treatment, gynecological examinations were performed. Both treatment groups had improvements in skin aging symptoms. The effects in the topical estriol group were superior. No hormonal side effects were noted either clinically or by hormone monitoring. The researchers concluded that local estrogen treatment appeared to be a promising new approach for anti-skin aging in perimenopausal females.

Estriol is a prescription drug in Canada, so you will need a doctor's prescription. A compounding pharmacy will make up the cream for you. Go to the Association of Compounding Pharmacies of Canada at www.acpcrx. org/ to find a compounding pharmacy near you. Because many doctors have never prescribed estriol before, here is the prescription so you can provide it to your doctor: 0.5 to 0.75 milligrams per dose. In the U.S., topical estriol is available in health food stores.

Do not forget to take a great multivitamin with minerals. Antioxidant vitamins and minerals like vitamins A, C, E, selenium and zinc are important at fighting factors that cause poor cell turnover which leads to brown spots, hyperpigmentation, redness, wrinkles and dry rough skin.

Now that we have learned about the food, nutritional supplements and topical agents that work in combination to give us the foundation for beautiful skin, let's discover all the exciting cosmetic rejuvenation treatments available.

How the Sun Can Damage Your Skin

Your skin increases the production of melanin in order to protect itself from the damaging effects of the sun. Melanin is the dark brown pigment in the top layer of skin that protects the deeper layers of skin from sun damage. The more melanin in the skin, the darker the skin appears. Sun exposure can cause an uneven increase in melanin production, resulting in irregular pigmentation of the skin. The sun can also cause a permanent increase in the small blood vessels, giving your skin a reddish appearance.

Solar lentigines, also known as liver spots or age spots, are brown, black or gray spots of increased pigmentation. These flat spots usually appear in areas that have had the most exposure to the sun such as the face, hands, arms and upper back. The number of age spots increase with repeated sun exposure and with advancing age.

The sun's UVA and UVB rays break down the skin's collagen and elastin fibers which lie in the deeper dermis of skin. Without the collagen and elastin fibers, the skin loses its strength and flexibility and vertical creases, deep wrinkles and loose or sagging skin occur.

Melasma, also known as the "mask of pregnancy," is a brown darkening of facial skin which results from a combination of factors, including exposure to sunlight and a disruption in female hormones. Melasma typically worsens after sun exposure.

Irregular areas of reddish-brown pigmentation known as poikiloderma, are commonly found on the neck and chest.

Actinic or solar keratoses are rough, scaly raised patches that range in color from dark pink to brown. These patches usually appear on the face, ears, lower arms and hands of fair-skinned people. If left untreated, actinic keratoses may progress to squamous cell carcinoma.

Lentigo maligna is a type of growth that begins as a dark flat spot and slowly darkens or enlarges. Lentigo maligna has the potential to develop into a melanoma. If you notice a change in the color, size or texture of a mole or if you develop a new skin growth that is troublesome, consult a health care professional immediately.

*Adapted from the Mayo Clinic, 2014.

CHAPTER 5: Cosmetic Treatments that Turn Back the Clock

More than ever, aging is a national health issue. For the first time in history in North America we have more women over the age of 50 than under the age of 50. With baby boomers now in their 50s and 60s, we are not only reconsidering our diet and health in general, but we are also exploring other ways to turn back the clock. At progressive clinics such as Dr. Braun's Vancouver Laser and Skin Care Centre, there are many options for facial rejuvenation and body contouring. What follows are non-surgical treatments that Dr. Martin Braun has found to be most effective.

DERMAL FILLERS

Dermal fillers are a great way to quickly bring a youthful appearance to the skin. There are many types of dermal fillers and they can be used to fill nasolabial folds, marionette lines, tear troughs and glabellar frown lines. Other uses include lip enhancement and cheek augmentation and correction of the jowls and nasal deformities.

The most commonly used non-permanent dermal filler contains hyaluronic acid. When hyaluronic acid is injected into the skin, it fills in areas that have lost collagen and it softens and hydrates the skin.

JUVÉDERM® FOR FULLER LIPS
Injectable Filler for Adding Volume to the Lips or the Face

The plump appearance of healthy skin is due to hyaluronic acid. This building block fills out the space between collagen and elastin fibers in the skin, holding in water and maintaining the skin's volume. In fact, one could argue that the hallmark of the aging face is volume loss which occurs due to the loss of fat and hyaluronic acid in the skin. As you age, levels of natural hyaluronic acid in the skin decrease with time, sun exposure and other lifestyle and environmental factors. This results in lines, furrows, wrinkles and thinner lips. Juvéderm® is the trade name for a hyaluronic acid filler for wrinkle correction and lip enhancement. Other brands of hyaluronic acid include Juvéderm Voluma®, Volbella®, Restalyne®, Perlane®, Teosyal® Ultimate and Belotero®.

How Juvéderm® Works

By injecting the skin with hyaluronic acid, we can mimic the effects of natural hyaluronic acid and produce the look and feel of hydrated skin. By filling depressions in the skin, wrinkles and folds are considerably softened and/or eliminated.

What to Expect

Hyaluronic acid is injected directly into the skin in tiny amounts using an ultra fine needle. Most hyaluronic acid brands are now formulated with lidocaine, a local anesthetic. If a patient wishes, local anesthetic can be used to make the entire procedure painless. This is particularly effective for lip enhancement. Many patients have had painful experiences with lip injections due to inadequate local anesthetic agents—there is no need to feel any pain at all. The procedure is convenient and the results are instantaneous. Juvéderm® is also available in an extra long lasting form called Voluma® and Volbella®.

Each procedure is customized. Most patients choose to have a follow up treatment between four to six months after the initial treatment. As the gel breaks down, water takes its place. When totally absorbed, the gel disappears unnoticed from the body.

Comparison to Other Hyaluronic Fillers

Juvéderm® is made from cross-linked hyaluronic acid fragments to form a very smooth syrup that is extremely unlikely to form any nodules or cause a skin reaction. In comparison, Restylane® and Perlane® use a stiffer formulation of hyaluronic acid. After years of use, Dr. Braun has found Juvéderm® to be the most natural filler available. Furthermore, if a patient does not like their "filler results," Juvéderm® can be dissolved with a natural enzyme within hours—the skin would be restored to its former state as it appeared prior to the injection.

There are four different fillers in the Juvéderm® family, each with their own level of viscosity: and Juvéderm® Ultra™, and Juvéderm® Ultra Plus™, Voluma®, and Volbella®. The type of filler used depends on the patient's needs and the specific area to be treated.

How to Minimize Bruising

Some patients will get a small bruise following a Juvéderm® injection. Although a tiny needle is used and every effort is undertaken to reduce the chance of bruising, it is possible to receive a bruise from an injection. If you are following our advice and taking skin nutrients, including a multi-vitamin that contains vitamins A, C, and E, the minerals zinc and selenium, and plant nutrients, you will find that bruising is limited. Ice can be applied before injections and should be applied immediately thereafter. If you are very prone to bruising, you will want to apply arnica homeopathic ointment after your treatment.

SCULPTRA® TREATMENTS

Derived from Fruit Acids for Restoring Youthful Facial Contours

Sculptra® is polylactic acid which is derived from fruit acids. When the micro-particles of polylactic acid are deposited deep under the skin by injection, they begin to stimulate collagen production as they are slowly broken down by the body. A natural, soft increase in dermal thickness begins to take shape within several weeks of injection. Sculptra® is especially beneficial for those with thin skin because it adds volume to facial tissue and restores shape and fullness to create youthful appearing facial contours.

What to Expect

Depending on the desired correction and the amount of material used at each session, patients normally choose to have three to four treatments. Over the course of four to six weeks, there is a gradual filling in the hollows, indentations and skin creases to restore youthful appearing facial contours. The improvements typically last several years and the procedure can be repeated as needed for maintenance.

The most common side effects are injection related, such as bruising and tenderness. A possible delayed side effect can be small bumps under the skin. These bumps may not be visible and you may notice them only when you press on the area. The bumps usually go away on their own, although occasionally visible bumps have been reported. Sculptra® was introduced in Europe in 1999, and many of the reported side effects of bumps under the skin occurred during its early use in the EU, Japan, and Australia. Sculptra® was only made available in Canada after 2006, and Canadian physicians and their patients have benefited with the knowledge gained by the European experience of injecting over 100,000 patients. Dr. Braun has found that the formation of bumps is quite rare in his experience.

PLATELET-RICH PLASMA (PRP)

Platelet-Rich Plasma Therapy – PRP Cosmetic Biophyl™ (hcPRP)

Many growth factors are involved in the repair and regeneration of soft tissue. The potential benefits of enhanced healing processes for skin depressions, wrinkles, acne scars, fine lines, crow's feet and collagen depletion have led to a recently widespread interest in the use of platelet-rich plasma therapy (also known as PRP or the Vampire Facelift®) for cosmetic improvement.

Although doctors have used PRP therapy since the mid-1990s to aid bone healing after spinal injury and soft tissue recovery following plastic surgery, it has only been more recently that the treatment has really come to the forefront. Since athletes such as Tiger Woods, Pittsburgh Steelers' Hines Ward, and L.A. Lakers' Kobe Bryant have been treated with PRP, people from around the world have been turning more and more to this type of therapy. In fact, according to the media, PRP injections in his elbow may have been the reason that Los Angeles Dodgers' pitcher Takashi Saito was able to return to the mound for the 2008 Major League Baseball playoffs.

How PRP Works

The allure of PRP is that it can provide an abundance of healing factors in the body's normal environment. Since platelets are responsible for healing and coagulation, as well as providing growth factors to stimulate tissue regeneration and repair, it makes sense to try to harness their power to stimulate collagen renewal in the skin. The theory behind PRP is that it may affect tissue healing via growth factors that are released after platelet degranulation.

HcPRP is highly concentrated platelet rich plasma therapy. Instead of using PRP from systems such as Selphyl®, that typically use a 2-8X concentration, the patented form of hcPRP involves injecting platelet-rich plasma in a concentration of 23-90X. The highly concentrated version of PRP is simple, safe and has no risk of any significant adverse effects because the patient is receiving his/her own platelet concentrate. Because of this natural benefit we inject hcPRP for the treatment of fine lines, wrinkles, folds and collagen loss. And although it can be injected into the same areas as common cosmetic fillers, it cannot compensate for major volume loss.

What to Expect

Following a consultation to determine if you are a suitable candidate and if you choose to have the treatment, a few vials of your own blood will be taken. The blood is spun in a centrifuge to separate the platelet-rich plasma from the other components. Then the concentrated platelets are injected into the area you wish to optimize in terms of benefits. In theory, the growth factors that the platelets secrete (not including human growth hormone) will spur tissue regeneration and the growth of collagen. The autologous nature (using your own blood) of PRP eliminates the risk of immune rejection or disease transmission.

Depending on the degree and extent of the wrinkles or folds, typically one to three treatment sessions are required. Injections are usually spaced four to six weeks apart. There is minimal discomfort at the time of injection because the area being injected is numbed before treatment begins. The area may feel slighty swollen and tender. Minimal discomfort may persist for two to five days. The regenerative repair process takes weeks to months. There have been no reported complications with PRP therapy.

DERMAL MICRO-NEEDLING

Dermal micro-rolling or skin needling encourages the production of collagen and elastin through the use of a dermal roller. Using a small hand-held rolling device, microsurgical needles are rolled over the skin which create tiny punctures in the epidermis and dermis. This procedure stimulates fibroblast cells to migrate to the injured site, produce collagen and elastin, and deposit new extra cellular matrix. Over time, this new matrix will cross-link and organize itself to fill in fine lines, wrinkles and scars. Growth factors are also released during this procedure resulting in firmer, toned and healthier skin. It is safe for all skin types and can be used on any area of the face, neck and body (except the lips and eyelids). Different sized needles are available and the size used depends on your needs:

- ▸ 0.25mm – Used to improve skin color and texture and to reduce fine lines and hyperpigmentation. This size is also used to increase the penetration of topical agents including vitamins A and C and cellulite creams.
- ▸ 0.5mm – For the reduction of wrinkles and light scarring.
- ▸ 1.0mm to 1.5mm – For stretch marks, cellulite and deep scarring.
- ▸ 2.0mm, 2.5mm, 3.0mm – For more severe or deep scars and wrinkles and the rejuvenation of damaged skin.

With a history dating back to ancient acupuncture techniques and meso-therapy, dermal rolling is supported by clinical studies as an effective non-surgical and non-ablative treatment for a variety of skin conditions when used regularly. Skin needling using needles up to 1.0mm can be used at home on a regular basis and as an adjunct treatment to in-office skin rejuvenation treatments. Platelet-rich plasma (PRP) therapy which we dis-cuss on page 66 can be used in a clinical setting along with dermal rolling.

How Dermal Rolling Works

As the needles are rolled over the skin, tiny punctures are created within the epidermis and dermis which encourages the production of collagen and elas-tin and the release of growth factors resulting in thicker, firmer and healthier skin. Despite the mental image of the process, it is not painful.

During the natural healing process, fibroblast cells—which are the cells that make collagen and elastin—migrate to the injured site and produce and deposit new extra cellular matrix. This new matrix cross-links and organizes itself and, over time, it will fill in any depressed scars, fine lines and wrinkles that are present; tighten and tone the skin; and reduce the signs of aging.

What to Expect

Dermal rolling stimulates collagen and elastin production and enhances the absorption of healing cosmetic agents. Forehead lines and frown lines are reduced, crow's feet and lip lines are softened and the appearance of wrin-kles, enlarged pores, scars, pigmentation, and sun damage are reduced.

Although skin needling has been demonstrated to be safe and effective, some individuals may experience slight pinkness and swelling in the skin initially. When using skin needling in combination with Retin-A or vitamin A topicals, a possible retinoid reaction (redness, flaking, burning or stinging) may occur due to the increase in vitamin A penetration. This is not harmful, just unpleasant. If irritation results, delay use of the dermal roller for a week or until the skin feels comfortable. Do not use a dermal roller on active acne, active rosacea, open wounds, infected areas, eczema, severe solar keratosis, skin cancer, raised moles or warts. If you are unsure about using your skin care product in conjunction with the dermal roller or for any other concerns, always consult a skin care professional.

Proper care and cleaning of the dermal roller is crucial to maintain its safety and effectiveness. Denture tablets (in water) may be used to clean the dermal roller. Denture tablets contain an enzyme cleanser which remove oils and reduce bacteria. In a plastic cup with a cotton pad placed at the bottom, use half of a denture tablet mixed with water, gently insert your roller and allow it to soak for 15 to 30 minutes. The dermal roller can also be cleaned with rubbing alcohol. Open the cleaning tray and place a white pad in the larger half of the tray. Fill the cleaning tray with rubbing alcohol and roll the roller into the pad with medium pressure. Leave the roller in the rubbing alcohol for 15 minutes and ensure that the roller drum is constantly wet with alcohol. Gently use your brush to clean away any skin cells. After cleaning, gently rinse with tap water, return the roller to the protective case and allow it to air-dry. Replace the case lid until the next use. Avoid dropping or resting your roller on a hard surface—it will bend the needles and your roller will no longer be safe to use. More importantly, never share your roller with another person.

MICRODERMABRASION
Exfoliation and Buffing for Aging Skin, Fine Lines, Scarring, Sun Damage and Wrinkles

Microdermabrasion helps to repair facial skin, which takes a beating from the sun and the effects of aging. Dr. Braun uses DermaSweep® Microdermabrasion. This treatment buffs and polishes the skin to achieve a healthy glow and help alleviate fine lines, pigmentation, acne and dull dry skin. It stimulates the production of skin cells and collagen. It is also popular for removing the rough skin of keratosis pilaris found on the upper arms and shoulders. It has proven to be a very popular, non-surgical cosmetic procedure with no downtime.

Conditions Treated
- Sun-damaged skin
- Fine lines and wrinkles
- Blackheads and whiteheads
- Acne prone skin
- Age spots

How Microdermabrasion Works

During a microdermabrasion treatment, nylon and silk bristles are moved across the skin with applied vacuum suction, resulting in a very gentle and controlled exfoliation of the skin. The treatment also removes dead surface cells and clears the pores. Over time, pigment fades away and surface irregularities, such as fine wrinkles and acne scars, begin to soften. The vacuum suction can be increased depending on the patient's tolerance for more aggressive blackhead clearance.

What to Expect

Treatment of the whole face takes 30 minutes. There is no pain. The area treated may be slightly pink for a day. For smooth skin, a little microdermabrasion goes a long way. Sloughing off the uppermost layer of the skin reveals a fresher, younger-looking face. Regular microdermabrasion is perfect for keeping superficial lines to a minimum. Skin products will penetrate better following microdermabrasion.

PHOTODYNAMIC THERAPY

Light Therapy for Skin Cancers, Photodamaged Skin and Acne

Photodynamic therapy (PDT) treats a combination of skin changes as well as significant sun damage using Levulan® and a light source to activate it. It is effective at treating pre-cancerous spots (actinic keratosis), acne, irregular pigmentation, improving skin texture and reducing pore size.

A PDT treatment session involves applying a clear photosensitizing solution called Levulan® to the skin. The patient feels nothing. The Levulan®, also known as aminolevulinic acid (ALA), is a completely natural compound present in all humans. ALA is a precursor of heme, used to make hemoglobin for our red blood cells. When ALA is applied topically to the skin, it is taken up preferentially by rapidly dividing cells, such as cancer cells or acne lesions. The Levulan® is taken up by these rapidly dividing cells. The ALA is typically left on the skin for 60 to 120 minutes to "incubate," and then "activated" with a special blue and red light. The skin appears red like a sunburn for a few days and the skin cancers peel off without any scars. Acne is also diminished and pores effaced.

What to Expect

PDT for skin rejuvenation usually consists of two to four treatments at three week intervals. Following the treatment, one can expect the skin to look mildly red or even sunburned. This redness can be expected to last for a few days.

The skin improves with a more even-colored tone, smaller pore size, smoother texture, and a more youthful, rejuvenated look. Reduction in over-all sun damage, as well as pre-cancerous lesions and potential early skin cancer changes can also be expected. PDT therapy is very effective for the face, neck, arms, chest, hands, torso and legs. Unlike liquid nitrogen for pre-cancerous lesions, PDT does not result in any white marks or scarring.

PHOTOREJUVENATION IPL

Intense Pulsed Light Targets Brown Spots and Red Vessels and Stimulates Collagen

In less than an hour, you can obtain more youthful and rejuvenated skin without any downtime. This is Lorna's favorite skin rejuvenation treatment. Intense pulsed light (IPL) laser treatments can reduce fine lines, blemishes and broken blood vessels; fade freckles and age spots; smooth rough skin; and improve skin tone and elasticity. Intense pulsed light can be used on the face, neck, arms, legs, back and chest. Intense pulsed light targets brown spots and red vessels and is the most popular laser facial treatment in the world.

Dr. Braun uses the Harmony® platform, one of the most versatile lasers in the world. The Harmony® uses advanced fluorescent technology, the next generation of intense pulsed light. During treatment, the IPL handpiece deliv-ers pulses of light to the treated area, which stimulates collagen produc-tion and fades capillaries and brown spots. This gives the skin an improved texture and allows it to reflect light better.

Other common names for this process are photorejuvenation, FotoFacial, or photofacial. All these treatments selectively target abnormal changes that develop with age and successfully improve fine lines, sun damage, age spots, the symptoms of rosacea, and numerous other facial flaws.

What to Expect

The entire area is scanned with the intense pulsed light. The area is usually treated with multiple passes with customized settings. The formation of new collagen results in the repair of sun damage and decreased fine lines. Pigment comes to the surface and sloughs off. Red and blue blood vessels typically fade. The skin looks younger and reflects light from its smooth surface—it glows. The results are gradual and cumulative, so that there is no startling change in the appearance of your face after just a single IPL treatment. People will likely remark on your more revitalized and youthful skin, but no one will know why! There is no downtime at all.

PIXEL® (FRACTIONAL SKIN RESURFACING)

Fractional Skin Resurfacing for Improved Texture, Tone and Minimizing Pores

Fractional skin resurfacing is commonly used to restore a youthful appearance to wrinkled, prematurely aged, or sun-damaged skin. While results can be excellent, traditional laser resurfacing can be painful and have extended downtime. In the past, people have sometimes been housebound and unable to return to work for weeks. However, a FDA-approved laser device called the Pixel® by Alma Lasers™, is designed to improve the quality and texture of the skin while it stimulates collagen regeneration—all without the discomfort or need for lengthy recuperation. Other examples of different fractional skin resurfacing devices are the Fraxel®, the Pearl and Sciton's ProFractional Therapy.™

How Laser Skin Resurfacing Works

Pixel® fractional skin resurfacing is based on the principle of microthermal treatment zones. The laser pulses create tiny holes in the skin, removing the epidermis and upper dermis. The treatment then triggers the body's natural healing process, stimulating the growth of new, healthy skin tissue from the edges of the microscopic hole. This targets small zones of the skin, leaving surrounding tissue untouched and intact. These large unaffected areas act as a reservoir for more effective and rapid tissue healing and collagen production. The end result: new, healthier, smoother tissue in place of skin imperfections with very fast healing times.

Any area of the skin can be treated that has surface irregularities including wrinkles, acne scars and stretch marks. Commonly treated areas include the face, neck, chest, hands and arms. Generally, treatment involves three to six sessions at three week intervals. The Pixel® is often bundled with other light-based therapies to achieve optimal results.

What to Expect

There is minimal discomfort during the treatment, and sensitive individuals are offered a topical anesthetic cream. The majority of patients do not require anything. Most commonly, clients feel some slight warmth with the pulse of the laser. Clients experience a sunburn-like sensation afterward (a few hours) that is easily neutralized with a gentle moisturizer.

Some flaking and redness can be experienced for two or three days with full recovery in about five to seven days. Your skin will look better within days following the treatment, and results steadily improve over the next few months.

LASER HAIR REMOVAL

Targeted Laser Energy to Reduce Unwanted Hair

Laser hair removal is the most common laser procedure in the world. Lasers produce a beam of highly concentrated light. The light emitted is well absorbed by the pigment or color located in the hair follicles. During laser hair removal, the laser pulses for a fraction of a second, allowing the hair to absorb the light and heat up. As it heats up, the hair shaft and bulb are damaged which significantly impedes the hair's ability to re-grow.

What to Expect

The result: A 50 to 80 percent (or better) reduction in unwanted hair. Hair is natural to your body and it grows in stages. At any given time, not all hairs are growing and lasers are most effective at targeting the growing hairs. In practice, no laser destroys all of the hair follicles. Some follicles are destroyed, while others are reduced to fine hairs or shocked into prolonged dormancy. Multiple treatments provide the best results.

Is Laser Hair Removal Permanent?

It is possible that with a sufficient number of treatments, true "permanent hair removal" can ultimately be achieved, but not for every single hair present in a given area. Be advised that the FDA has cleared these lasers for "permanent hair reduction," and not "permanent hair removal," which is advertised by many clinics.

Age, ethnicity, weight, metabolism, medication and hormones all play a role in the location, resilience and thickness of hair. It is difficult if not impossible to predict how many treatments each individual will require to achieve the best long-term benefits. Experience to date with laser hair reduction suggests that the hair reduction achieved may be permanent, but an honest and reputable physician cannot guarantee such an outcome. Dr. Braun has published the world's longest peer-reviewed follow-up study on laser hair removal. Eighteen months after five treatments with the LightSheer® or Soprano® lasers, patients had an average reduction of 90 percent of the hairs on their legs.

THERMAGE® CPT
Radiofrequency for Enhancing Facial Contours and Skin Tightening
Unlike facelifts, Thermage® CPT helps to achieve a younger look without incisions or downtime. The Thermage® CPT procedure reduces the signs of aging skin by actually tightening the underlying tissue. It is currently used for non-surgical brow lifts and the non-surgical tightening of facial wrinkles on the forehead, around the eyes, the mid and lower face, and the neck. It is best suited in cases where the skin is only slightly lax or only a small degree of sagging occurs.

With the touch of a sophisticated treatment tip to the skin, Thermage® CPT uses radiofrequency energy. The top layers of the skin are protected with a cooling spray while the radiofrequency energy heats up the collagen in the lower layers. This deep volumetric heating causes the skin to tighten and new collagen to grow, producing a more youthful appearance.

What to Expect
The treatment can take up to two hours. Each time treatment is delivered, there is an immediate cooling sensation followed by a brief hot sensation, followed again by a cool sensation. Each person is unique and results are variable. We recommend patients rest the day of the procedure. Some people choose to go back to work on the following day. Results appear gradually in two weeks to six months.

ACCENT® XL
Contour the Body and Conquer Cellulite
Accent® XL radiofrequency therapy can bring back a fresh, firm and youthful appearance. Facial and body contouring through the production of collagen and improved skin surface texture is possible with the Accent® XL device. Using selective dermal heating, this device non-invasively tightens loose skin, promotes healthy collagen production and improves body shape.

The Accent® XL can be used to treat loose, sagging skin anywhere on the body including the face, abdomen, thighs, chest and upper arms. It can also be used to improve and diminish the appearance of cellulite. Although other radiofrequency devices on the market are used for the improvement of cellulite, the Accent® XL is by far the strongest.

How Accent® XL Works

During treatment, the Accent® XL device precisely heats an area of the inner layer of skin while simultaneously cooling the outer layer of skin. As the inner layer is heated, a natural reaction occurs, promoting the creation of new collagen. In the case of cellulite, it changes the shape of fat cells and shrinks and remodels the connective tissue that forms this unsightly condition.

Depending on the size of the treated area, the procedure may take up to 45 minutes. The heating action causes the deep structures of the skin to tighten. Many patients notice an improvement in their body silhouette after just one session.

What to Expect

Most people tolerate Accent® XL treatments well and have little or no discomfort. Patients often describe the sensation as a "warm massage." Following treatment, you can immediately resume all routine activities. You may notice slight redness from the heating effect, which should disappear in a few hours. Generally, three to six treatments at two- to four-week intervals are recommended. Accent® XL treatments can be combined with Lipodissolve, an alternative to liposuction for resistant fat deposits.

COOLSCULPTING® BY ZELTIQ®

Say Goodbye to Stubborn Fat Deposits

Cryolipolysis is a FDA-approved process that uses precisely controlled cooling methods to reduce fatty tissue, particularly around the flanks and love handles. Designed to target only your fat cells, this process does not harm your skin or other tissue. As a result of the cooling process, fat cells are destroyed. Your body's natural cleansing process removes those fat cells for gradual fat reduction over time.

How CoolSculpting® Works

You will not require any anesthesia or incisions. During your treatment, the CoolSculpting® device is applied to the targeted area to destroy unwanted fat cells without any harm to the adjacent tissues or your skin. During the next two to four months, the body naturally cleanses itself of the treated fat cells.

What to Expect

Because this treatment does not involve anesthesia or incisions, you do not have to plan for any downtime or recovery period. Some patients experience redness and mild bruising for a short time after the procedure. Multiple treatments produce the best results.

LIPODISSOLVE AND MESOTHERAPY
Injectable Fat-dissolving Substances Target Cellulite and Localized Fat Deposits

Body contouring without extensive surgery is possible. Lipodissolve and mesotherapy treatments consist of small injections of a natural lecithin and enzyme combination that is highly effective for dissolving the small, stubborn fat deposits that resist diet and exercise. The treatments consist of a series of small injections into the target areas of localized fat. Injection lipolysis (another name for Lipodissolve) will also reduce or eliminate unsightly lipomas, which are smooth, round benign tumors of fatty tissue.

What to Expect

Results are usually obtained in three to eight treatments. It is a quick office procedure and any side effects such as bruising, itching and soreness are minimal and temporary. Most patients lose one to three inches around their waistline.

Over the past 20 years, doctors in South America, South Africa and Europe have successfully used mesotherapy procedures on hundreds of thousands of patients. However, some non-medical spas and practitioners with little experience have had difficulties with these injections. It is imperative that you seek treatment from a well-established medical clinic with a long track record.

Treatment Areas

The areas that respond best to Lipodissolve treatment—in those who are not obese—are stubborn fat deposits that resist further reduction after diet and exercise. These include double chins, the abdomen, love handles, the back of the arms, thigh saddlebags, knees, and wings (the area on the back, just beside the armpits). Lipodissolve has also been shown to improve and smooth out the skin and shrink lipomas. Lipodissolve may be used in conjunction with Accent® RF and/or Zeltiq® CoolSculpting® for non-surgical fat reduction. Lipodissolve treatments are especially effective for reducing fat along the jawline. Lipodissolve can be used in conjunction with the Accent® RF to tighten the facial skin along the jawline in those who wish to avoid a traditional facelift with liposuction.

LEG VEIN TREATMENTS
Non-Surgical Foam Treatments for Varicose Veins and Spider Veins

If you have symptoms such as pain, aching and swelling in your legs or even restless legs at night, you may be suffering from an underlying venous disease with incompetent veins. In the past, incompetent veins had to be surgically remove or "stripped." This is painful and leaves scars. Now there is a better choice: ultrasound-guided foam chemoablation. For incompetent veins, a foam-like medication is injected while simultaneously monitoring the veins on an ultrasound screen. This allows for accurate placement of the medication into the diseased veins that often leak and feed into the bulging surface veins. The foam that is injected into the veins causes the vein walls to collapse. Compression stockings are then used for a few days to make sure that the vein walls stay collapsed. There are no wraps or bandages. There is no surgical incision.

Spider veins can be treated with traditional sclerotherapy and/or lasers. Sclerotherapy is a simple procedure whereby the visible veins are injected with a sclerosing solution, which causes them to collapse and fade from view. If sclerotherapy hasn't worked for you in the past, it may be that you have underlying incompetent veins that you cannot see because they can only be found with ultrasonic mapping of the lower limbs. If the underlying incompetent veins are closed with foam using an ultrasound, visible sclerotherapy should work much better on the remaining superficial tiny spider veins.

Lasers allow delivery of a precise dosage of energy to each vein. The light energy is absorbed by the blood vessels but not the surrounding tissue. This heat absorption causes a coagulation of the blood vessel, which is subsequently absorbed by the body.

What to Expect

To begin treatment, the entire vein anatomy of the lower limbs is mapped out with a sophisticated ultrasound. The causes of the varicose veins and spider veins are identified, and the problem is treated first at the source, and then followed up with treatment of the varicose veins. By treating the problem in this fashion, the long-term success is very high and the risks are very few. There is no surgical risk with anesthesia, no downtime or dressings, and very little discomfort. Multiple treatments may be required to reduce the unsightly appearance.

We recommend being reasonable in your expectations. If you have extensive vein issues that need to be addressed, it is often better to take care of them in more than one visit in order to minimize the exposure to discomfort. You will likely have some bruising. Pigmentation changes may persist for a while, and it is dependent on your body's ability to clear the tissue. Discomfort is to be expected, but it is generally not significant and does not impair usual activities. You will have better results if you wear support stockings after leg procedures. Bruises may be covered with makeup.

We recommend you take Veinsmart after your treatment to improve the appearance of varicose or spider veins. See page 119 to learn more about Veinsmart.

BOTOX®: REAL RESULTS FOR THE AGING FACE

We are sure that the discoverer of the botulinum toxin way back in 1897 would not have believed that this toxin could be purified and used on millions of people for conditions such as excessive sweating, chronic migraines, crossed eyes in children as well as wrinkles.

Botulinum toxin type-A (BTX-A) was first used in the 1980s to treat strabismus or "crossed eyes," a condition in which the eyes are not aligned properly. BTX-A's full potential was not realized until 1989, when a plastic surgeon in California by the name of Dr. Richard Clark published the first documented use of BTX-A for cosmetic use in *Plastic and Reconstructive Surgery*. There are now three brands of BTX-A in Canada: Botox®, Xeomin® and Dysport®.

How Does It Work?

BTX-A, commonly known as Botox®, acts on the nerve endings in muscles to prevent muscle fibers from contracting. By reducing these contractions, Botox® can temporarily reduce expression lines like the ones on your forehead or between your brows. It has been over 25 years since the first Botox® cosmetic injections were done for unsightly frown lines between the eyebrows. Due to the fact that the long-term safety of Botox® has now become clinically established with tens of millions of men and women, Botox® treatments have become the number one cosmetic procedure in the world. How did the Botox® phenomenon develop to become a regular part of grooming for millions? The answer is quite simple: Almost anyone can be treated and those that are treated absolutely love the relaxed, smooth look.

Since Botox® injections target wrinkles that result from excessive muscle contraction, people with lines around the eyes or a frown that they would like to soften are all suitable candidates. One ten minute treatment—a few tiny injections—blocks the nerve impulses and relaxes the muscle. As the muscle relaxes, the wrinkle overlying the muscle is smoothed away.

Considering that Botox® only relaxes the muscle beneath the line at the injection site, the treatment has no effect on sensory nerves or other elements of facial expression which allows for a normal feeling in the treated areas. Most people will have a more relaxed, calm, and friendlier appearance a few days after treatment. The benefits of Botox® usually last for at least four months. After several treatments, improvements appear to last longer.

If treatment is performed properly, Botox® is quick, relatively painless and has no downtime. Some individuals may experience rare side effects such as bruising or the dreaded "droopy eyelid." Any side effects that do develop are temporary and usually mild. Botox® can be combined with high-tech skin laser procedures, chemical peels, microdermabrasion and fillers. The combined approach produces an even better result as can be seen in Figure 1.

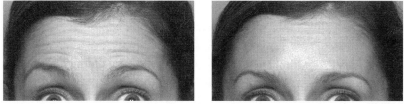

Figure 1

Botox® is commonly used in the following areas:
1. Horizontal forehead lines. Look in the mirror and lift your eyebrows. Some foreheads resemble a plowed field. A good practitioner will put in just enough Botox® to soften those forehead lines without completely losing the ability to lift the brow. People communicate with their brows, and if the forehead does not move at all, the appearance is one of fatigue or the "deadpan" expression that everyone dreads.
2. Around the eyes. As we age, the wind, sun, time, and laughter all create wrinkles around the eyes called "crow's feet." Some patients say they have "earned those lines," but that is like saying you also deserve middle-age spread. Six to twelve units of Botox® around the eyes can often result in a more wide-eyed, alert and attractive appearance. Botox® can

also lift the brow, and for most women, the brow is everything. Women like to have more "plateau" for their eye makup, and some have called the skin below the lateral brow the most valuable real estate on a woman's face.

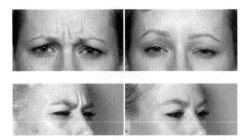

Figure 2

3. Around the mouth. Vertical lip lines are like cellulite, the bane of every woman's existence. The appearance of these lines, as well as their progression, can be improved by the judicious use of a few units of Botox® around the mouth. Botox® injections into the upper lip result in increased lip show with a more averted upper lip border. As we age, we also develop a downturn of the lateral edges of the mouth. This is called a "mouth frown" and it portrays a bitter expression. Who doesn't like the Mona Lisa smile? Botox® can help your smile muscles lift the corners of your mouth when one injects the opposing muscles that pull it down. We can't do anything about gravity, but we can weaken the muscles that pull your face down. Why assist the gravitational effects on our face when we can diminish downward pull on our face?

4. Botox® can also be injected in the point of the chin, softening a dimpled chin appearance. Studies have also shown that if one also enhances the lip with a filler at the same time as the Botox® treatment, the filler will last longer.

5. Lower facial reshaping and temporomandibular joint (TMJ) dysfunction due to enlarged masseter muscles. An enlarged masseter muscle causes a broad face with "chipmunk cheeks." Asian females in particular, prefer the appearance of a heart-shaped or V-shaped face because a broad face is masculinizing. The Koreans pioneered the use of Botox® to shrink the masseter muscle in order to produce a pleasing V-shape. This cosmetic treatment led to the use of Botox® to alleviate the discomfort of clenching and grinding teeth, which is not uncommon at night for many people. Clenching and grinding is known as bruxism, and this leads to wearing down of the molars and even cracked teeth, temporomandibular joint

(TMJ) pain and headaches. The relief of this tension is profound for those who suffer from bruxism and wear night guards prescribed by their dentist.

6. The neck and décolleté are often neglected because women feel that there is little that can be done to improve these areas, which is far from the truth. Horizontal neck lines, vertical muscle bands running down the neck and those V-shaped grooves on the sun exposed upper chests of women can all be softened with Botox®.

Botox® has also been used with increasing frequency by doctors during the last two decades for more and more medical conditions. One of the most exciting observations by patients undergoing Botox® injections in their frown areas was that they experienced fewer headaches, which led to FDA and Health Canada approval of Botox® for the treatment of chronic migraines. In fact, Dr. Braun's experience is that over 80 percent of his patients experience blissful breaks from migraines and tension headaches.

Botox® is also used to treat excessive sweating (hyperhidrosis) of the underarms, palms of the hands and the feet. These patients suffer in silence, frequently avoiding social situations and clothing that shows their profuse perspiration. Botox® can also do amazing things for cervical and laryngeal spasms (uncontrolled spasms of the shoulders, neck, larynx, voice box or limbs) following a stroke, multiple sclerosis and brain and spinal cord injuries.

The use of Botox® continues to expand. Botox® was recently investigated for alleviating prostate enlargement in men, a condition that affects more than half of men over the age of 75. It works by relaxing the prostate gland and improving urine flow. Botox® can also be used to treat those individuals with an overactive bladder. Another recent study showed that Botox® helped patients suffering from tinnitus or ringing in the ears, as well as trigeminal neuralgia.

SUMMARY

In this section, we have described many of the most advanced and popular skin rejuvenation treatments. For more information on cosmetic treatments that we have not addressed, please visit www.vancouverlaser.com.

The next chapter is probably the one that you have been waiting for, if you have not already skipped ahead. In "Beauty SOS," we shape everything that we have discussed so far into a variety of integrated solutions for your common skin concerns. Just like we are seeing excellent advances in medicine by combining conventional and complementary treatments, so too can we successfully blend nutritional medicine and advanced dermatology. Why not combine the best of both to achieve optimal results?

TREATMENT OPTION	WHAT IT DOES
Dermal fillers	Injectable fillers for adding volume to the lips or the face.
Sculptra® treatments	Injections derived from fruit acids for restoring youthful facial contours.
Platelet-rich plasma (PRP) therapy	Use your own platelets to enhance healing, stimulate tissue regeneration and repair the skin.
Dermal micro-needling (skin needling)	Promotes the production of elastin and collagen in the skin using microsurgical needles.
Microdermabrasion	Exfoliation for aging skin, fine lines, scarring, sun damage and blackheads.
Photodynamic therapy	Light therapy for skin cancers, photodamaged skin and acne.
Photorejuvenation IPL	Intense pulsed light targets brown spots and red vessels and stimulates collagen production.
Fractional skin resurfacing	Improves texture and tone and minimizes pores.
Laser hair removal	Targeted laser energy to reduce unwanted hair.
Thermage® CPT	Radiofrequency for enhancing facial contours and skin tightening.
Accent® XL	Contour the body and conquer cellulite.
CoolSculpting®/Cryolipolysis	Reduce fatty tissue deposits, especially around flanks and love handles, using precisely controlled cooling methods.
Lipodissolve and mesotherapy	Injectable fat-dissolving substances target cellulite and localized fat deposits.
Leg vein treatments	Non-surgical foam treatments for varicose veins and spider veins.
Botox®	Injections of BTX-A to target wrinkles that result from excessive muscle contraction.

CHAPTER 6: Beauty SOS

Now that you have learned the skin basics, and some of the best foods and supplements to support your skin from within, what's your current beauty SOS? Whatever challenge your skin is facing, even if it is just the effects of premature aging, this chapter is designed to provide you with simple solutions that work fast for healthier, more youthful-looking skin.

We will discuss the most common skin issues, everything from acne to wrinkles. We will start with suggested nutritional supplements for each condition, followed by dermatological treatment options from Dr. Braun, and finish with the additional lifestyle tips for best results.

ACNE AND BLEMISHES

During puberty, peri-menopause and menopause, sebaceous (oil) glands become more active. Pores can become clogged with sebum, dried skin and bacteria, causing the skin to erupt into pimples, red blotches and sometimes inflamed and infected abscesses. Acne normally appears on the face, shoulders, scalp, upper arms and legs, and upper chest and back. More than 40 percent of teens seek treatment from a specialist for their acne condition.

Hormonal acne break-outs tend to occur during ovulation or the week before menstruation. In those women with hormonally induced acne, when the ovary releases the egg, it often is not able to completely release it. When this occurs, androgens (male hormones) are secreted in excess and women develop acne. To correct hormonal acne, many doctors prescribe birth control pills to stop ovulation. (Today we have 12-year-olds on birth control pills to control acne.) Nutritional supplements can normalize ovulation and eliminate the problem at the source.

Symptoms

There are various types of skin lesions: a *papule* is a round bump that may be invisible but makes the skin feel rough like sandpaper. A *comedo* occurs when an oil follicle becomes plugged with oil, dead skin, tiny hairs or bacteria. An open comedo is known as a blackhead, and a closed comedo is commonly referred to as a whitehead. The temporary red or pink spot after an acne lesion has healed is referred to as a *macule*, and several together contribute to the appearance of inflammation associated with acne. A *nodule* is another dome-shaped lesion similar to a papule, but it extends deeper into the skin, causing the destruction of tissues that leads to scarring. Nodules and cysts can be painful, severely inflamed and also affect deeper skin layers.

Causes

While food choices have been hotly debated as a cause of acne for years, research out of the University of Colorado confirms that a diet high in refined carbohydrates permanently boosts insulin and thus promotes acne. According to Dr. Loren Cordain, sustained high insulin levels elevate hormone levels, stimulating the production of oil that leads to clogged pores, bacterial growth and acne. High-glycemic foods such as breads, cakes, sugars and soda are major culprits in acne. Although acne is epidemic in our society, it is virtually unknown in New Guinea and the Amazon where diets focus on fruits and vegetables. Those with acne should be conscious of foods that aggravate the condition. Acne is also associated with low stomach acidity, suggesting incomplete food breakdown and imbalances in the digestive tract.

With the shift between male hormones and female hormones during the menstrual cycle, acne lesions change. Synthetic progestins and estrogens used for menopausal symptoms, DHEA supplements, endometriosis, polycystic ovarian syndrome and estrogen dominance have been linked to acne. Other drugs such as corticosteroids, anabolic steroids, iodides and bromides are also known to cause acne, as are cosmetics that block pores.

PRESCRIPTION FOR HEALTH

Nutrient	Dosage	Action
Multivitamin with minerals (contains no iron); Multismart	As directed; should contain the following nutrients: Vitamin A 1250 IU	Reduces sebum production and promotes smooth, clear skin
	Beta carotene 7500 IU Folic acid 500 mcg P-5-P (vitamin B6) 30 mg	Facilitates the breakdown of excess hormones
	Vitamin B3 15 mg, along with other B vitamins Vitamin D 500 IU	Promotes healing of the skin
	Vitamin E 100 IU	Acts as an antioxidant and encourages tissue repair
	Zinc 7.5 mg In one study, 135 mg of zinc daily was as effective as 750 mg daily tetracycline without side effects.	Essential for healthy immune function
	Chromium polynicotinate 100 mcg	Improves glucose tolerance and fatty acid metabolism
	Selenomethionine 50 mcg	To enhance glutathione and fight bacteria
GLA Skin Oil	2 tsp daily	Helps fight acne
Cala-Q Plus containing coenzyme Q10	2 softgels per day	Helps heal skin
Estrosmart	2 capsules per day containing: Indole-3-carbinol 150 mg Sulforaphane 200 mcg D-glucarate 150 mg Curcumin 50 mg Rosemary 25 mg DIM 50 mg Green tea extract 100 mg	Balances hormones Supports healthy ovulation Within two menstrual cycles, acne will clear and PMS and period problems will ease.
Probiotic Plus	2 capsules daily. Each capsule contains: 2.5 billion active cells of BB536 Bifidobacterium 250 mg of whole cranberry extract	Improves intestinal flora (especially important if you have taken antibiotics for a condition)

Nutrient	Dosage	Action
Balance-T	Drink Balance-T throughout the day	Detoxifies the liver
Digestive enzymes	1 or 2 capsules with meals	Aids digestion

General Considerations/Options by Dr. Braun:

Supplement your skin care regimen with exfoliating alpha hydroxy acids (glycolic, mandelic, lactic acid) and beta hydroxy acids (salicylic acid). These products remove dead cells on the skin surface and reduce oiliness. Everyone with acne should also be applying a vitamin A (retinol) cream to their skin at night. Unfortunately, many manufacturers do not disclose the amount of retinol in their products, and these producers put miniscule amounts in their products. Only use a retinol product if the manufacturer puts the amount of retinol on the label. Like the hydroxy acids, retinol can be irritating. If your skin is sensitive, use these products sparingly or use 0.05% topical retinol every second or third night.

Technology that will help control acne includes microdermabrasion (for exfoliation), blue light therapy or IPL (to kill bacteria) and Accent® RF to reduce oil production. Photodynamic therapy does all three at once.

Additional Health Tips to Enhance Healing:

▸ Wash your face gently with warm water and an irritant-free cleanser. Avoid scrubbing, which can stimulate sebum production. Do not use makeup that will clog pores.

▸ Do not pick at acne, as this can lead to infection.

▸ If you have gas, bloating, indigestion or constipation, you might have low stomach acid. Take a supplement with betaine hydrochloride or digestive enzymes to improve digestion.

▸ Avoid the use of antibiotics which may have little effect on acne and can cause Candida yeast overgrowth and vaginal infections that will worsen acne symptoms in the long term and may have little effect on acne.

▸ Focus on a diet rich in fruits and vegetables along with 25 g of fiber daily to help naturally eliminate estrogen. Avoid foods that you know will aggravate the condition.

▸ Treat constipation. Holding days of toxic waste increases the amount of toxins excreted by the skin.

ALOPECIA (HAIR LOSS)

Alopecia simply means hair loss. Male pattern baldness is the most common form of alopecia. Inflammation, psoriasis, and fungal infections of the scalp are also associated with hair loss.

Alopecia areata is an autoimmune disorder whereby a person's immune system prevents hair follicles from producing hair fiber. Men and women are affected equally with this autoimmune disorder. According to the American Autoimmune Related Diseases Association, it is estimated that roughly 2 million people have some variation of alopecia. The condition can strike at any time, and may begin as early as childhood. This section, although focusing on autoimmune hair loss, provides treatments for all hair loss.

Symptoms

Alopecia areata, the mildest form of the condition, is marked by hair loss that is partial or patchy on the scalp and other parts of the body. In a more severe form called alopecia totalis, all facial and/or scalp hair may be lost. The most extreme case is called alopecia universalis and the entire body loses its hair. Sometimes hair loss is permanent; at other times, it may grow back. Those with alopecia may notice other symptoms such as brittle nails or onychogryposis, a condition where the nails have thickened with increased curvature. Often alopecia is seen with other autoimmune disorders, particularly Hashimoto's thyroiditis, lupus, Addison's disease, vitiligo and diabetes.

Causes

Organ-specific autoantibodies are increased in those persons with alopecia areata. Although no specific autoantibody has been found specific to the hair follicles, researchers believe alopecia is an autoimmune disorder because of genetic predisposition; there is usually the presence of other autoimmune disorders and a positive response to corticosteroid treatment.

Nutritional deficiencies in biotin and zinc have been found to contribute to alopecia. Many women experience alopecia postpartum, during menopause, and as a result of taking birth control pills, which suggest a hormone connection.

Testosterone supplements have been associated with increasing hair loss. Testosterone is converted to dihydrotestosterone (DHT). DHT is known to inhibit the growth and development of hair in the follicle. As well, high-fat diets cause an increase in free testosterone and as such are also implicated in hair loss. People with high blood levels of insulin-like growth factor-1 (IGF-1) have higher rates of baldness. There is an interplay between androgen hormones, insulin and other hormones in the body. One factor alone does not seem to promote alopecia.

Research has shown that smoking may also increase hair loss by increasing the production of androgen hormones. It is also thought that smoking has a direct effect on hair follicles by killing the hair fiber-making cells.

Several research papers have suggested that alopecia in men may be related to heart disease. Researchers believe that increased rates of heart disease in those with alopecia may be due to elevated cholesterol. Cholesterol is converted into androgen hormones in the body.

In women hair loss has been associated with low iron levels. When iron stores returned to normal, hair re-growth occurred. Conversely, iron overload has also been shown to cause hair loss, especially in men. Hemochromatosis is a genetic disease whereby the individual's body stops breaking down and removing iron from the bloodstream, which promotes hair loss.

Tamoxifen, a drug used in treatment for breast cancer, has been demonstrated to cause alopecia. Withdrawal of the drug stops the condition; however, hair may or may not grow back. Chemotherapeutic agents may also cause hair loss.

PRESCRIPTION FOR HEALTH

Nutrient	Dosage	Action
Multivitamin with minerals (contains no iron); Multismart	As directed; should contain the following nutrients: Vitamin A 1250 IU Beta carotene 7500 IU Folic acid 500 mcg P-5-P (vitamin B6) 30 mg Vitamin B3 15 mg, along with other B vitamins Vitamin D 500 IU Vitamin E 100 IU Zinc 7.5 mg Chromium polynicotinate 100 mcg Selenomethionine 50 mcg	Improves circulation, protects against free radical damage, essential for healthy immune function and is anti-inflammatory.
GLA Skin Oil	1-2 tsp daily	Reduces inflammation and restores skin function

Nutrient	Dosage	Action
Ironsmart	1-3 tsp daily	Important for circulation and oxygen transport to cells. Low ferritin is the leading cause of hair loss in women today. Can also be a factor in fatigue, hair loss, peeling finger-nails, heart palpitations, poor concentration, heavy periods and pale skin.
Thyrosmart	If you have low thyroid, take two capsules at breakfast containing: Potassium iodide 100 mcg. Ensure your total daily iodine from all sources does not exceed 300 – 400 mcg.	Iodine's only role in the body is to make thyroid hormones. Too little causes impaired thyroid function; too much iodine interferes with the thyroid's ability to make thyroid hormones.
	Tyrosine (amino acid) 500 mg	A key component in the function of the thyroid gland
	Sensoril® Ashwagandha 125 mg	Increases T4 thyroid hormone. Acts directly on the thyroid gland.
	Commiphora mukul extract (Gugguls) 120 mg	Enhances the conversion of T4 to the more active T3. Works synergistically with ashwagandha directly on the thyroid gland.
	Pantothenic acid 100 mg	Supports the adrenal glands; increases energy; helps you handle stress better.
	Copper 500 mcg	Support for the thyroid gland
	Manganese 500 mcg	Support for the thyroid gland
Collagen Plus	Mix 10 drops daily in juice. Each drop contains: Silicic acid 1 mg	Collagen makes hair elastic so there is less breakage and less hair in your brush.

Nutrient	Dosage	Action
	Biotin 50 mcg	Silicic acid and biotin for shiny, thick and strong hair.
Adrenasmart	1 to 2 capsules per day. Each capsule contains: Rhodiola 100 mg (*Rhodiola rosea*)	Helps reduce the effects of stress, is anti-aging and regulates the heart by increasing oxygen utilization
	Suma 100 mg (*Pfaffia paniculata*)	A regenerative tonic used for nervous, reproductive, hormonal and digestive disorders
	Sensoril® Ashwagandha 62.5 mg (*Withania somnifera*)	Improves energy, supports the immune system, is antioxidant and anti-inflammatory, improves sexual performance. It is also used to aid the conversion of T4 to T3 thyroid hormone. Normalizes reactions to physical and mental stress, enhances energy, protects against environmental pollutants, regulates blood sugar, protects the liver and adrenals.
	Schizandra berries 80 mg (*Schizandra chinensis*)	For insomnia and nervousness supports the liver and improves physical endurance

General Considerations/Options by Dr. Braun:

Red light-emitting diodes (LED) have been shown to increase hair growth on the scalp. There are even hats and helmets that contain red LEDs to promote hair growth. One example is the iGROW helmet available at http://www.igrowlaser.com. An individual can wear this at any time, making it a convenient way to stimulate hair growth.

Additional Health Tips to Enhance Healing:

▶ The main cause of hair loss in women is hypothyroidism, commonly called low thyroid. Have your thyroid hormones tested. You may still experience symptoms even if your results are not enough to be clinically diagnosed. Supplement with Thyrosmart and read *An A-Z Woman's Guide to Vibrant Health* by Lorna or visit www.hormonehelp.com for more thyroid-support suggestions.

▶ Have your iron levels (hemoglobin and ferritin) checked. Low levels of iron and conversely, high levels of iron in the blood are associated with hair loss. If you are iron deficient, take Ironsmart. If you have excess iron, donate blood.

▶ Diet is also important to support healthy iron levels. Start the day with a protein-rich breakfast (an egg, a chicken breast, a protein shake, or protein powder in yogurt) and eat protein and greens at every meal thereafter.

▶ Hair loss can be caused by oral medications. These include drugs for cholesterol reduction, Parkinson's, arthritis, ulcer drugs, antidepressants, beta-blockers for high blood pressure, epileptic anticonvulsants and steroids.

▶ An estimated 2 percent of North Americans are affected by alopecia areata, an autoimmune skin condition that causes partial or patchy hair loss on the scalp and other parts of the body. This occurs when your immune system accidentally attacks hair follicles and hair growth is arrested. Consult a naturopathic doctor and/or a dermatologist if you suspect auto-immune disease.

BLACKHEADS, WHITEHEADS AND MILIA

Dermatologists refer to blackheads and whiteheads as comedones, but any-one who has them refers to them as undesirable. These bumps or cysts are caused by a blockage of pores or hair follicles. A blackhead looks like dirt because dead protein (keratin) has blocked the pore and has oxidized to a darker color. Whiteheads are rooted in the dermis under the epidermis, a deeper kind of blemish that is more likely to cause scarring if you pick at it. Whiteheads are often mistaken for milia, which look like tiny white bumps. Although milia are also closed-over keratin plugs like whiteheads, they are not considered to be acne or linked to bacteria or oil. Aging and slower cell turnover cause milia, which generally start to show up in your thirties.

Regular exfoliation is recommended to combat these three pore-blocking problems. Try a physical exfoliation such as a home-based scrub or a micro-dermabrasion treatment at a professional clinic once a week. See page 69 for more information on microdermabrasion. Chemical exfoliation methods include the use of salicylic or glycolic acids. According to Dr. Braun, many women exacerbate the problem by using moisturizers that are too heavy for their skin type. Women with "sensitive skin" or "dry skin" simply have unhealthy skin that has become accustomed to heavy, daily moisturizer use. Their natural skin barrier that prevents water loss has been compromised, and pores have been blocked, leading to milia and larger pores.

BROWN SPOTS (MELASMA OR "SUN SPOTS")

Brown spots, also known as melasma or sun spots, are a common skin condition that causes brown discoloration above the upper lip and on the cheeks and forehead. Brownish spots or patches often develop on the female face, particularly in young mothers and in women taking contraceptives. It is very common in pregnant women and is often referred to as "the mask of pregnancy." Oxidative stress also contributes to the overproduction of skin pigment, and exposure to sunlight greatly contributes to further oxidative stress.

PRESCRIPTION FOR HEALTH

Nutrient	Dosage	Action
Multivitamin with minerals (contains no iron); Multismart	As directed; should contain the following nutrients: Vitamin A 1250 IU	Promotes smooth, clear skin
	Beta carotene 7500 IU Folic acid 500 mcg P-5-P (vitamin B6) 30 mg	Facilitates the breakdown of excess hormones
	Vitamin B3 15 mg, along with other B vitamins Vitamin D 500 IU	Promotes healing of the skin
	Vitamin E 100 IU	Acts as an antioxidant and encourages tissue repair
	Zinc 7.5 mg	Essential for healthy immune function
	Chromium polynicotinate 100 mcg	Improves glucose tolerance and fatty acid metabolism
	Selenomethionine 50 mcg	To enhance glutathione and fight bacteria
GLA Skin Oil	1-2 tsp daily	Restores skin function

Nutrient	Dosage	Action
Cala-Q Plus containing Coenzyme Q10	2 softgels per day	Helps heal skin
Estrosmart	2 capsules per day containing: Indole-3-carbinol 150 mg Sulforaphane 200 mcg D-glucarate 150 mg Curcumin 50 mg Rosemary 25 mg DIM 50 mg Green tea extract 100 mg	Balances hormones
Probiotic Plus	2 capsules daily. Each capsule contains: 2.5 billion active cells of BB536 Bifidobacterium 250 mg of whole cranberry extract	Improves intestinal flora (especially important if you have taken antibiotics for a condition)
Balance-T	Drink Balance-T throughout the day	Detoxifies the liver
Digestive enzymes	1 or 2 capsules with meals	Aids digestion

General Considerations/Options by Dr. Braun:

There is no cure for melasma, also known as "the mask of pregnancy." However, it is possible to treat and control the condition by daily use of sulforaphane, a safe sunscreen and multiple different skin-brightening agents. These include kojic acid, phytic acid, and other alpha hydroxy acids as well as arbutin, licorice, retinol and vitamin C. Laser treatments and advanced depigmentation masks used in a clinical setting can produce some very good results.

Additional Health Tips to Enhance Healing:

▸ Be careful of overexposure to the sun. Even though melasma has its roots in hormonal imbalance, this condition is exacerbated by the sun. Wear protective clothing, a hat and a broad-spectrum sunscreen whenever you are outside.

▸ Focus on a diet rich in fruits and vegetables along with 25 g of fiber daily to help naturally eliminate estrogen.

▸ Eliminate hormone disruptors in your home and personal care products.

Read Lorna's book *A Smart Woman's Guide to Hormones* to learn where all the hormone disrupting agents are in your cosmetics, food and environment.

▸ Use a sulforaphane ointment, not the lotion, to promote cellular repair and reduce sun damage. Lorna has used this to reverse brown spots but you have to commit to using it every day.

▸ Use a non-toxic, broad-spectrum sunscreen. Go to the Environmental Working Group's Skin Deep® Cosmetics Database at www.ewg.org/skindeep. Lorna's favorite brands are Badger and Aubrey Organics. Dr. Braun likes Colorescience® minerals and Jane Iredale pressed minerals, especially for oily or acne prone skin. The high zinc powder content in these products renders the skin surface inhospitable to P. acne, the bacterium that causes almost all acne. Another unique sunscreen is ZO Skin Health Oclipse®, which contains natural melanin. When ultraviolet light hits our skin, it makes melanin for protection. So it makes sense to put natural melanin on the skin to help protect it from the sun's harmful UVB rays.

▸ Taking fatty acids like GLA Skin Oil will also help naturally build melanin in the skin.

CELLULITE

You have most likely heard of "orange-peel skin," a phrase used to describe how cellulite looks and feels. Under your epidermis and dermis are three layers of fat, and cellulite forms in the first subcutaneous fat layer called the hypodermis. Connective tissue holds the fat chambers in this area. Cellulite is mostly fat, but simply losing weight will not always eliminate the orange-peel appearance. Cellulite develops in steps. It starts with damage to your lymphatic drainage system caused by a poor diet and digestion, not enough protein in the diet, a lack of exercise or excessive activity, an accumulation of toxins, repeated weight loss and weight gain, hormone imbalance, aging and/or a toxic liver.

A female's fat under the skin is separated by fibrous bands (septae) which compartmentalize the fat, much like an egg crate container or ice cube tray. As fat is gained and lost over time, some compartments shrink while others expand, leading to an irregular surface. Cellulite affects almost all women.

Cellulite Is Caused By:

- A diet devoid of vegetables
- Fat gain
- Yo-yo dieting (repeated weight loss and gain)
- High sugar consumption
- Liver congestion caused by toxin overload
- Inadequate consumption of protein, which causes water retention
- Lack of vitamins and minerals
- Poor digestion
- Poor insulin regulation in the body due to high-carbohydrate diet
- Lack of exercise
- Excessive or repetitive exercise of the legs without exercising other areas
- Excessive caffeine and alcohol consumption
- Smoking, which impairs circulation
- Stress, which leads to high cortisol levels
- Pregnancy (because of its increased pressure on the lymphatic and venous systems and because of weight gain)
- Adrenal exhaustion, causing a craving for salt, which promotes excess water retention
- Untreated food allergies
- Estrogen imbalance, especially during menopause or perimenopause
- Constipation, hemorrhoids, and varicose veins which put pressure on the lymphatic system
- Repeated air travel, which impedes the flow of lymph and blood

Estrogen and Cellulite

Estrogen has a direct effect on the metabolism of skin and hair, changes in body composition, and alterations of subcutaneous fat distribution throughout your life. Estrogen dominance creates a host of health problems including endometriosis, uterine fibroids, fibrocystic breasts, breast cancer, ovarian cysts, heavy periods, estrogen belly, low thyroid, and fat deposits. Excess estrogen is thought to be the culprit that causes cellulite to build up around the fat cells and restrict lymphatic drainage and blood flow.

At menopause, the decline in estrogen promotes cellulite. It seems that too much or too little estrogen can create problems with connective tissue and can cause skin aging, lack of elasticity in the skin, and sagging skin. An excess of estrogen in the younger years, followed by erratic estrogen levels (highs and lows) at menopause, can cause cellulite to become extreme in the years after menopause.

Estrogen Mimickers

Environmental estrogens, also called estrogen mimickers and xenoestrogens (pronounced "zeno estrogens"), further exacerbate the estrogen overload. These toxic estrogens are found in common everyday substances—plastics, pesticide-laden foods, deodorants, nail polish, cosmetics, foods containing dioxins (meat, milk, eggs and fish), glues and adhesives—and they disrupt your estrogen balance, which leads to weight gain, poor thyroid function and cellulite.

Fortunately, keeping your estrogens healthy and balanced is possible even when you are exposed to a daily onslaught of environmental estrogens. And here's how:

- Eat only organic foods because pesticide-laden fruits and vegetables are the main source of xenoestrogens.
- Take Estrosmart every day. Estrosmart contains nutrients such as indole-3-carbinol, calcium D-glucarate, green tea extract, diindolylmethane (DIM), rosemary leaf extract, curcumin and sulforaphane. These nutrients balance your hormones and detoxify and eliminate carcinogenic estrogens.
- Do not microwave foods in plastic; use only glass or ceramic containers. Estrogen mimickers, such as bisphenol-A, lurk in plastics.
- Detoxification is vital for cellulite reduction. Epsom salt baths and infared saunas are excellent for improving the appearance of cellulite.

More Cellulite Busting Tips

If you are overweight, losing weight is important, but don't be discouraged if your cellulite is still visible after you have lost 10 lbs (4.5 kgs). The fat accumulation within cellulite is usually the last fat to be eliminated. Read *A Smart Woman's Guide to Weight Loss*. This program is perfect for reducing cellulite and keeping it off. Good, clean sources of protein, plenty of low glycemic index vegetables, and essential fatty acids will help remove all of these stubborn deposits. A diet deficient in protein causes water retention, reduced cellular repair, and cellulite.

PRESCRIPTION FOR HEALTH

Nutrient	Dosage	Action
Multivitamin with minerals (contains no iron); Multismart	As directed; should contain the following nutrients: Vitamin A 1250 IU	Promotes smooth, clear skin
	Beta carotene 7500 IU Folic acid 500 mcg P-5-P (vitamin B6) 30 mg	Facilitates the breakdown of excess hormones
	Vitamin B3 15 mg, along along with other B vitamins Vitamin D 500 IU	Promotes healing of the skin
	Vitamin E 100 IU	Acts as an antioxidant and encourages tissue repair
	Zinc 7.5 mg	Essential for healthy immune function
	Chromium polynicotinate 100 mcg	Improves glucose tolerance and fatty acid metabolism
	Selenomethionine 50 mcg	To enhance glutathione and fight bacteria
Estrosmart	2-4 capsules daily. Each 2 capsules contain: Indole-3-carbinol 150 mg Sulforaphane 200 mcg D-glucarate 150 mg Curcumin 50 mg Rosemary 25 mg DIM 50 mg Green tea extract 100 mg	Balances hormones; detoxifies excess estrogens; prevents estrogens from converting into cancer-causing estrogens.
CLA Plus with Green Tea Extract	6 softgels daily. Each softgel contains: Conjugated linoleic acid (CLA from safflower oil) 730 mg Camellia sinensis (Green tea extract) 113.3 mg	Aids weight loss, increases lean muscle, accelerates fat loss, and controls blood sugar. A powerful antioxidant.
Glucosmart	1-2 capsules daily. Each capsule contains: D-chiro-inositol (Chirositol™) 600 mg Chromium (picolinate) 2.2 mcg	Fights belly fat and elevated hormones, reduces appetite, improves serotonin and helps control blood sugar.

Nutrient	Dosage	Action
Collagen Plus	10 drops daily in juice. Each drop contains: Silicic acid 1 mg Biotin 50 mcg	Required to maintain the normal growth, development and integrity of healthy bones, joints, hair, nails and connective tissue. Cellulite is linked to a silicon deficiency in the cells' protein matrix surrounding these areas.
Protein powder	1-2 scoops daily in a smoothie or at breakfast	Required for muscle repair and formation; a good source of EFAs

Detoxification Baths

Detoxification baths increase blood flow to the skin's surface and open the pores, thereby encouraging perspiration and toxin elimination. Start the baths slowly at five minutes, working your way up to 30 minutes. Take only one a week, then two, and so on, as you may experience adverse effects, especially if your toxic load is great. If you experience dizziness, headaches, fatigue, nausea, or weakness during a bath, get out of the tub. Next time, bathe for a shorter period in cooler water. To take a detoxification bath, fill the tub with water as hot as you can tolerate. Drink at least two or three glasses of purified water before, during and after your bath. You may also wish to accelerate detoxification by adding 1 cup (250 mL) of Epsom salts to a regular bath and gradually increase the amount to 4 cups (1 L) per tub.

Sweating is Good for You!

Heavy perspiration from exercise and saunas aids elimination of toxins from your body. A detoxification sauna should be preceded by twenty minutes of exercise and followed by a cleansing shower. You can lose up to 4 cups (1 L) of water during a twenty-minute sauna, so be sure to replace lost fluids.

Dry Brushing Improves Circulation

Use a skin brush made of soft, natural, non-abrasive bristles. Do up to five minutes of long strokes over every area of your body, always moving toward your heart. For example, start at your feet and brush toward your heart. Then start with your buttocks, stomach and chest and brush toward your heart.

Lymphatic Drainage Speeds Results

Your lymphatic system circulates lymph fluid throughout your body. That fluid carries toxic wastes and bacteria to the lymph nodes, where the toxins are engulfed and destroyed by cells of the immune system. It is especially important that the lymphatic system remains decongested. Lymphatic massage can be done daily to facilitate detoxification.

Exercise—even just rebounding for twenty minutes a day—is another way to revive a sluggish lymphatic system and improve circulation. Please read *A Smart Woman's Guide to Weight Loss* by Lorna for more information.

Topical Treatments: Cellusmart

Cellusmart contains green coffee bean extract which has been shown to cause fat cell lipolysis and smooth the orange peel look of the skin. Green coffee extract also works on alpha receptors. Researchers recently discovered that the fat within cellulite tissue responds very well to the inhibition of the alpha receptors. Alpha receptors are found on the surface of fat cells within cellulite tissue. Once inhibited, these alpha receptors allow fat to exit from the cellulite tissue and enter the bloodstream to be burned by other tissues. The resulting fat reduction minimizes skin dimpling and wrinkling and creates a smoother, more attractive look in the affected area.

Researchers working in this field have discovered that certain plants contain natural substances that directly inhibit these alpha receptors, release the fatty deposits and reverse cellulite appearance to an appreciable degree. Cellusmart by Lorna Vanderhaeghe contains green coffee bean extract and caffeine. Women should also use Estrosmart in conjunction with applying Cellusmart topical cream morning and night, massaging it well into the skin.

An anti-cellulite cream alone will not break down stubborn fat deposits, but good food, exercise and detoxification, combined with a good-quality topical cellulite product that promotes blood flow and metabolizes fats, will speed up the process. Other ingredients offering promising results include retinol, gotu kola, caffeine and butcher's broom.

Additional Options/Comments by Dr. Braun:

There is a plethora of technologies used to treat cellulite that can be classified as:

1. Rollers assisted by vacuum suction that knead the skin and fat. Endermologie® from France is an example of this technology.
2. Piston and vibration devices that "hammer" the skin: e.g. VibraSlim®.
3. Radiofrequency (RF) heating devices. These devices cause deep dermal

heating to contract collagen. Examples include Thermage® and Accent® RF. Some devices combine RF with rollers, such as the Velashape® or Velasmooth®.

4. Infrared LED or laser devices. These devices use red light wavelengths and claim to result in "leaky" fat cells that cause the fat to shrink, e.g. the Lipolite®.

5. Ultrasound (focused and non-focused). These devices heat the collagen and shrink it using ultrasound energy. Examples are the Liposonix®, Accent® Ultra and Ultrasonix devices. All of these devices require multiple treatment sessions in order to achieve a decent aesthetic result. In addition, the aging process never stops, so ongoing maintenance is required to maintain the improvement. Many practitioners combine mesotherapy with these technologies. Mesotherapy consists of injecting minute amounts of vitamins, minerals, and natural fat-dissolving enzymes into the cellulite to reduce the subcutaneous fat. Very nice results with skin smoothening are possible.

DARK CIRCLES UNDER THE EYES

PRESCRIPTION FOR HEALTH

Nutrient	Dosage	Action
Multivitamin with minerals (contains no iron); Multismart	As directed; should contain the following nutrients: Vitamin A 1250 IU	Promotes smooth, clear skin
	Beta carotene 7500 IU Folic acid 500 mcg P-5-P (vitamin B6) 30 mg Vitamin B3 15 mg, along with other B vitamins	
	Vitamin D 500 IU	Promotes healing of the skin
	Vitamin E 100 IU	Acts as an antioxidant and encourages tissue repair
	Zinc 7.5 mg	Essential for healthy immune function
	Chromium polynicotinate 100 mcg	Improves glucose tolerance and fatty acid metabolism
	Selenomethionine 50 mcg	To enhance glutathione and fight bacteria

Nutrient	Dosage	Action
GLA Skin Oil	1-2 tsp daily	Reduces inflammation and restores skin function
Ironsmart	1-3 tsp daily if you have anemia or low iron, which can contribute to dark under-eye circles. Have your iron levels tested.	Important for circulation and oxygen transport to cells. Low iron can also be a factor in fatigue, hair loss, peeling fingernails, heart palpitations, poor concentration, heavy periods and pale skin.

General Considerations/Options by Dr. Braun:

Dark circles under the eyes are one of the most difficult cosmetic concerns to treat. Often, the cause is multifactorial. There may be excessive pigment which can be lightened with IPL (intense pulsed light) as well as various fading creams. There may also be a component of vascular congestion due to multiple blue veins and pooling of blood. This can also be improved with what is called an Nd-YAG laser, which targets the blue venous blood. Finally, the dark color is exacerbated by the tear trough effect. As we age, the lower eye bag expands outwards, forming a trough effect along the lower lid that accentuates any dark circles. This trough can be filled with natural, biodegradable fillers to improve the appearance.

Additional Health Tips to Enhance Healing:

▶ Have your iron levels checked. Iron is so important to your overall health that even mild deficiencies can affect your appearance with dark blue/black circles under the eyes, which are a telltale sign of iron deficiency and iron deficiency anemia.

▶ Test your adrenal gland function. Rest for five minutes and then take your blood pressure. Stand up and immediately take another blood pressure reading. If the reading is lower when you are standing than when you are resting, you can suspect decreased adrenal gland function.

▶ Fatigue can exacerbate dark under-eye circles. If you are under stress resulting in fatigue and sleeplessness, practice anti-stress strategies. Breathing is a powerful de-stressing tool. Several times per day, breathe in through your nose and fill your lungs with air until your abdomen rises. Then slowly exhale from your mouth until your lungs empty. Repeat five times.

▶ Puffiness can make under-eye circles look darker. Sometimes, the parasympathetic nervous system is not able to drain and circulate fluids properly during sleep. Congestion of the veins under the eyes results. Get eight hours of sleep every night and try to sleep until 7:30 in the morning.

▶ To reduce puffiness, apply a used cold teabag to the eyes for 20 minutes.

▶ Drink water—8 to 10 glasses of pure, clean, filtered water every day.

What Kind of Iron Do I Need?

One in four women suffers from low iron or iron deficiency anemia. Women are more susceptible than men to iron deficiency anemia due to blood loss during their monthly menstrual cycle. Yet more than 57 percent of women do not get enough iron from their diet. Women require up to 20 mg of iron daily during the childbearing years, but most get less than 10 mg per day from food and often it is poorly absorbed. Simply taking 10 mg of elemental iron per day will solve this.

Traditional doctor prescribed iron like ferrous fumerate or ferrous sulphate are difficult to absorb and hard on the digestive system. Iron can irritate the intestinal walls and cause pain, cramping, diarrhea, constipation and black stools. Thankfully, there is a new form of iron that works fast to raise hemoglobin and ferritin without any side effects.

Ironsmart iron is a liposomal form of iron where each molecule of iron is wrapped in a liposomal bubble that allows the iron to pass through the high-acid stomach environment and go directly to the small intestine, where it is absorbed directly by the receptor for iron. Results from a recent study showed that the absorption of Ironsmart liposomal iron, tested two hours after oral administration, was five times greater than ferrous fumarate. After 12 hours, the absorption of Ironsmart liposomal iron was far higher than all other forms of iron. Ironsmart is available in two forms: a delicious, caramel flavored liquid iron and a vegetarian capsule. Ironsmart raises ferritin and hemoglobin quickly and it does not cause constipation.

ECZEMA

Eczema is an allergic condition whereby abnormalities in the immune system promote an overproduction of inflammatory and allergic reactions in the skin. This leads to poor resistance to skin bacteria and viruses. It is estimated that 10 percent of North Americans suffer from eczema. It is common in infants and toddlers and often appears when the child is teething or after immunizations. There are five types of eczema: atopic (allergic), infantile seborrheic, adult seborrheic, occupational irritant contact and allergic contact dermatitis.

Symptoms

Eczema is intensely itchy and the skin may be flaky, thick, scaly, weeping or crusting, or it may change in color. The skin inflammation commonly appears on the wrists, ankles, face, and the creases of the knees, ears, between the fingers and on the elbows. Skin thickening often occurs after much scratching and rubbing, and bacterial or viral infections are also common.

Causes

Children are more likely to develop eczema if there is a history of asthma, eczema or hayfever in the family. Triggers include stress, infections and climate changes. Stress is a major factor in adult eczema flare-ups. Those with eczema often have allergies, proven by allergy tests and elevated IgE levels, as well as a family history of the condition. Common allergens are food additives and preservatives, milk, eggs, wheat, soy, tomatoes, oranges and peanuts. Eczema can be the result of other conditions such as Candida albicans, leaky gut syndrome and a lack of stomach acid. Those with eczema often have poor digestion, which increases allergic reactions. Severe essential fatty acid deficiency is also associated with the development of eczema, with the skin unable to hold moisture properly. In occupational irritant contact and allergic contact dermatitis, exposure to environmental allergens such as metal alloys in zippers and jewelry, cosmetics, perfumes, rubber, latex and poison ivy are the source of the problem. Infantile seborrhea is more commonly known as cradle cap and adult seborrhea is red, dry, flaky skin that may also appear as mild dandruff.

PRESCRIPTION FOR HEALTH

Nutrient	Dosage	Action
Celadrin Super Rich Skin Therapy Cream	Apply to the skin twice per day if the skin is not broken	Powerful anti-inflammatory; inhibits immune factors that promote inflammation of the skin
Multivitamin with minerals (contains no iron); Multismart	As directed; should contain the following nutrients: Vitamin A 1250 IU	Promotes smooth, clear skin

Nutrient	Dosage	Action
	Vitamin D 500 IU	Promotes healing of the skin
	Vitamin E 100 IU	Acts as an antioxidant and encourages tissue repair
	Zinc 7.5 mg	Essential for healthy immune function
	Chromium polynicotinate 100 mcg	Improves glucose tolerance and fatty acid metabolism
	Selenomethionine 50 mcg	To enhance glutathione and fight bacteria
GLA Skin Oil	Adults: 4-6 tsp per day Children: 1-2 tsp per day	Reduces inflammation in the skin; improves moisture retention
Quercetin	500 mg, three times daily	Anti-inflammatory and anti-allergy; halts histamine release
Digestive enzymes	1 or 2 capsules with meals	Aids digestion

General Considerations/Options by Dr. Braun:

Patients with eczema should always use moisturizers on their skin that are simple, non-irritating, and free of artificial fragrances, colorants, and preservatives especially parabens. Oatmeal baths are soothing, but remaining too long in a hot bath will dry the skin out.

Additional Health Tips to Enhance Healing:

▶ Eczema is often linked to food allergies or intolerance. Start a diet diary; write down everything that you eat to see if there is any correlation to your symptoms. Ask for a referral to an allergy specialist and get tested for possible triggers. Once you know what you are allergic to, avoid those allergens.

▶ Have your thyroid checked. Low thyroid function impairs the immune system causing increased inflammation.

▶ Do not take immune boosters because they enhance macrophage function and increase inflammation in the cells of the skin thereby aggravating eczema.

▶ Eat seven to ten half-cup servings of vegetables every day. If you haven't been eating raw veggies regularly, start with steamed vegetables; they will be easier on your digestive system.

▶ Take GLA Skin Oil essential fatty acids orally and also apply GLA to the skin. Make sure you do a spot test before applying it to eczema to ensure you do not have a reaction the first time you use it.

▶ Eat plenty of cold-water fish (salmon, herring, halibut, mackerel) and fatty acid-rich seed and nut oils; these foods help heal eczema.

▶ Avoid deep-fried foods, meat, food that is high in sugar and other refined carbohydrates (like white bread), caffeine, alcohol and dairy products.

▶ Use Celadrin Super Rich Skin Therapy Cream topically to soothe and heal inflamed skin.

▶ Use hypoallergenic laundry detergents and rinse your bedding, towels and clothing twice to eliminate detergent residue. Do not use fabric softeners or dryer sheets; these are often a source of skin irritation and allergy.

▶ Drink water—8 to 10 glasses of pure, clean, filtered water every day.

▶ Long term use of strong cortisone ointments can cause serious side effects and skin thinning. They should not be used continuously. Avoid using them on small children, and determine underlying allergies quickly before chronic skin inflammation occurs.

PSORIASIS

Psoriasis is a very common skin condition characterized by the rapid production of skin cells, leading to a congestion of cells on the skin's surface. The normal life cycle of skin cells is 28 days, but cells produced by psoriasis mature up to a thousand times faster than those of healthy skin. Psoriasis can also cause an inflammatory form of arthritis called psoriatic arthritis. More than 7 million North Americans have psoriasis, with its onset generally in the late twenties. According to The National Psoriasis Foundation, 56 million hours of productivity are lost annually in the U.S. due to psoriasis. Treatment costs US$1.6 to $3.2 billion every year.

Symptoms

Raised patches of red with white flakes or scales appear on the torso, elbows, knees, legs, back, arms and scalp. When it is in the scalp, psoriasis can promote hair loss. In some people, the nails may become dull, pitted or ridged and may separate from the nail bed. Psoriasis fluctuates between periods of inflammation and remission and is categorized as mild, moderate or severe. If the skin becomes too badly damaged, there can be fluid loss, bacterial infection and an inability to regulate temperature. Approximately 400 people die every year from psoriasis. There are psychological ramifications to psoriasis as well, as people may feel shame, embarrassment, social rejection and anger due to a lack of understanding on the part of their peers. Arthritis similar to rheumatoid arthritis, called psoriatic arthritis, is sometimes present in those with psoriasis and it is very difficult to treat. There is pain, morning stiffness, swelling, reduced range of motion, pitting of the nails, tiredness and redness in the eye (conjunctivitis). In severe cases, it can lead to deformity of the joints and spine. Difficult to diagnose in people with subtle symptoms, it is believed that 10 to 30 percent of those with psoriasis will also develop psoriatic arthritis. It usually appears between 30 and 50 years of age.

Causes

The cause of psoriasis is unknown, but two theories have emerged: it is an autoimmune disorder, or it is caused by a bacterial "superantigen." Either way, there is a glitch in the immune system that tells the body to produce more skin cells. The immune system is often hyper-stimulated, promoting inflammatory cytokines in the skin cells. It may also be that the immune system, after a viral or bacterial infection, becomes primed to attack the skin. Common triggers for psoriasis flare-ups are poor diet, incomplete protein digestion, a diet including excessive animal fat, bowel toxemia, impaired liver function or heavy alcohol consumption. Other triggers are reactions to medication, stress, sunburn, illness, injury, nerves or surgery.

PRESCRIPTION FOR HEALTH

Nutrient	Dosage	Action
Multivitamin with minerals (contains no iron); Multismart	As directed; should contain the following nutrients: Vitamin A 1250 IU	Promotes smooth, clear skin
	Beta carotene 7500 IU Folic acid 500 mcg P-5-P (vitamin B6) 30 mg	Facilitates the breakdown of excess hormones
	Vitamin B3 15 mg, along with other B vitamins Vitamin D 500 IU	Promotes healing of the skin
	Vitamin E 100 IU	Acts as an antioxidant and encourages tissue repair
	Zinc 7.5 mg	Essential for healthy immune function

Nutrient	Dosage	Action
	Chromium polynicotinate 100 mcg Selenomethionine 50 mcg	Improves glucose tolerance and fatty acid metabolism To enhance glutathione and fight bacteria
Celadrin Super Rich Skin Therapy Cream	Apply to the skin twice per day if the skin is not broken	Powerful anti-inflammatory; inhibits immune factors that promote inflammation of the skin
High-lignan ground flax seeds	1-2 teaspoons per day	Improves bowel function; reduces bowel toxicity
Vitamin D	1,000-2,000 IU daily	Reduces immune factors that promote inflammation of the skin
GLA Skin Oil	Adults: 4-6 tsp per day Children: 1-2 tsp daily	Reduces inflammation in the skin; improves moisture retention
Comfrey or stinging nettle tea	Apply to the head daily as a rinse	Loosens scales; heals scalp psoriasis

General Considerations/Options by Dr. Braun:

Psoriasis responds to sunlight. Although it is safer to avoid prolonged sun exposure in order to reduce the risk of sunburn and skin cancer, people with psoriasis will experience an improvement in their symptoms with sunlight. It is also important to keep the skin moisturized.

Additional Health Tips to Enhance Healing:

▶ Avoid saturated fats; they promote flare-ups of psoriasis. Consume a diet that emphasizes natural, whole foods such as legumes, fresh fruit and vegetables, fish, healthy fats and oils, and nuts and seeds. Opt for foods high in vitamin E and vitamin C. Avoid animal meat and choose cold-water fish such as salmon, halibut and mackerel instead.

▶ Stress reduction is essential. Thirty-nine percent of those with psoriasis report that stress initiates the disease. If you are under stress, take Adrena-smart as directed.

▶ Eliminate caffeine, sugar and alcohol.

- ▸ Do not take immune boosters that enhance macrophages as this can cause inflammation in the skin.
- ▸ Get a little sun. Psoriasis seems to abate during the summer months and that is thought to be a result of UV radiation.
- ▸ Allergies and food sensitivities are common for those with psoriasis. Ask for a referral to an allergy specialist and get tested for possible triggers. Environmental allergies should be tested as well.
- ▸ Try natural alternatives to corticosteroid creams such as Celadrin Super Rich Skin Therapy Cream or GLA Skin Oil by Lorna, or salves with capsaicin, licorice and chamomile. Lorna recommends Botanical Therapeutics' shampoo and conditioner for those with scalp psoriasis.

Celadrin and Psoriasis

A double-blind, placebo-controlled study using Celadrin cream for the treatment of psoriasis was performed over a 14-day period. Patients were asked to apply the cream to the affected area twice a day. The initial severity of skin scales, patchiness, redness, dryness, cracked and raised skin were recorded. Then after 7 and 14 days, each patient visited the dermatologist who evaluated their skin. Each patient experienced a two level improvement based on the 6-point Liker scale (0 = no improvement, 5 = significant improvement). This small pilot study found that those persons using Celadrin cream experienced a measurable improvement in their psoriasis. Celadrin Super Rich Skin Therapy Cream also helps those with eczema, rosacea and other skin conditions by halting inflammation and healing the skin.

ROSACEA

A chronic skin disorder causing acne-like breakouts, broken blood vessels and redness mostly on the cheeks and nose, rosacea generally strikes people after the age of 30 and it affects three times more women than men. If the problem is not addressed, it can cause permanent damage to the skin. Although the cause of rosacea is not known, there are a number of triggers specific to each individual that aggravate the condition: smoking, hot liquids, spicy foods, stress, caffeine, excessive alcohol, ginkgo biloba, menopausal flushing, lack of stomach acid or the digestive enzyme lipase, infection, exposure to sunlight and food and environmental allergies.

PRESCRIPTION FOR HEALTH

Nutrient	Dosage	Action
Multivitamin with minerals (contains no iron); Multismart	As directed; should contain the following nutrients: Vitamin A 1250 IU	Reduces sebum production and promotes smooth, clear skin
	Beta carotene 7500 IU Folic acid 500 mcg P-5-P (vitamin B6) 30 mg	Facilitates the breakdown of excess hormones
	Vitamin B3 15 mg, along with other B vitamins Vitamin D 500 IU	Promotes healing of the skin
	Vitamin E 100 IU	Acts as an antioxidant and encourages tissue repair
	Zinc 7.5 mg In one study, 135 mg of zinc daily was as effective as 750 mg daily tetracycline without side effects.	Essential for healthy immune function
	Chromium polynicotinate 100 mcg Selenomethionine 50 mcg	Improves glucose tolerance and fatty acid metabolism To enhance glutathione and fight bacteria
Celadrin Super Rich Skin Therapy Cream	Apply to the skin twice per day if the skin is not broken	Powerful anti-inflammatory; inhibits immune factors that promote inflammation of the skin
Vitamin C	500-1,000 mg daily	Enhances collagen formation
Vitamin D	1,000-2,000 IU daily	Reduces immune factors that promote inflammation of the skin
Cala-Q Plus	2 softgels daily	Controls inflammatory factors; ensures adequate EFA levels; maintains skin integrity

Nutrient	Dosage	Action
GLA Skin Oil	Adults: 4-6 tsp per day Children: 1-2 tsp per day	Reduces inflammation in the skin; improves moisture retention
Pancreatic enzymes	500 mg before meals	Improves digestion and metabolism of fats

General Considerations/Options by Dr. Braun:

Patients with rosacea almost always have skin that is sensitive to many skin care products. They should always try one product at a time, and initially apply it every second day to determine their tolerance to the product. Products with low levels of retinol, coffeeberry and green tea are often tolerable for rosacea patients if introduced slowly to their skin care regimen. The chronic redness and broken capillaries seen in rosacea can also be diminished with intense pulsed light (IPL) and/or a pulse dye laser. Several treatments are often required to fade the red spots. In addition to fading the redness, IPL also results in the formation of new collagen in the skin. This improves the ruddiness often associated with rosacea.

Additional Health Tips to Enhance Healing:

▶ Eliminate sugar, dairy and hydrogenated fats. This is essential to halting rosacea.

▶ Alcohol is a very strong trigger for rosacea, so reduce or eliminate alcohol.

▶ Drink at least eight to 10 glasses of pure, filtered water daily. Water flushes out toxins and encourages efficient elimination.

▶ Eat foods that encourage healthy liver function such as artichokes, rhubarb, Chinese white radish, black radish, apples and rolled oats.

▶ Do not consume hot food and drinks. Let them cool to room temperature first.

▶ Allergies are also implicated in rosacea. Ask for a referral to an allergy specialist and get tested for possible food and environmental triggers.

▶ Antibiotics have been effectively used to treat rosacea in some cases. If using antibiotics, take probiotic supplements as well.

▶ Apply Celadrin Super Rich Skin Therapy Cream and GLA Skin Oil daily to help halt inflammation and heal the skin.

▶ Use all natural, mineral-based makeup and choose unscented soaps, cleansers, shampoos and detergents. Avoid perfumes and scented body sprays.

▶ Flushing is provoked by higher temperatures, so avoid conditions that are too hot or too warm, such as you would find in saunas, hot tubs and hot baths.

SCARS

There are many different kinds of scars. They can appear either white (hypopigmentation) or dark (hyperpigmentation). They can be indented like a "box car" which is frequently seen after chicken pox, or pitted like an "ice pick" which often occurs in the case of acne. Or they can be firm, which is the result of abnormally constructed collagen due to skin trauma or surgery. In a normal skin matrix, collagen is woven together horizontally, but scar tissue forms fast and chaotically, resulting in a disorganized knot of tissue. A hypertropic scar is raised and firm, the same size of the original wound. Lastly, keloid scars grow beyond the original wound and often occur on the earlobes or the central chest.

PRESCRIPTION FOR HEALTH

Nutrient	Dosage	Action
Multivitamin with minerals (contains no iron); Multismart	As directed; should contain the following nutrients: Vitamin A 1250 IU	Promotes smooth, clear skin
	Beta carotene 7500 IU Folic acid 500 mcg P-5-P (vitamin B6) 30 mg	Facilitates the breakdown of excess hormones
	Vitamin B3 15 mg, along with other B vitamins Vitamin D 500 IU	Promotes healing of the skin
	Vitamin E 100 IU	Acts as an antioxidant and encourages tissue repair
	Zinc 7.5 mg	Essential for healthy immune function
	Chromium polynicotinate 100 mcg	Improves glucose tolerance and fatty acid metabolism
	Selenomethionine 50 mcg	To enhance glutathione and fight bacteria
Collagen Plus	Mix 10 drops daily in juice. Each drop contains: Silicic acid 1 mg Biotin 50 mcg	Important for building and retaining a healthy matrix. Silicic acid and biotin help build collagen.

Nutrient	Dosage	Action
GLA Skin Oil	Adults: 4-6 tsp per day Children: 1-2 tsp daily Each tsp contains GLA 500 mg	Reduces inflammation in the skin; improves moisture retention
Vitamin C	1,000-2,000 mg daily with bioflavonoids	Important for proper collagen formation; reduces inflammation; strengthens immunity; antioxidant properties
Cala-Q Plus	2 softgels daily	Controls inflammatory factors; maintains skin integrity
Probiotic Plus	2 capsules daily. Each capsule contains: 2.5 billion active cells of BB536 Bifidobacterium 250 mg of whole cranberry extract	Supports immune function; prevents infection; restores healthy bowel function and replenishes good bacteria after antibiotic use

General Considerations/Options by Dr. Braun:

Intense pulsed light (IPL) can help fade red or brown color in scars. Fractional resurfacing is a laser technique which burns tiny holes into the skin. This is a controlled injury designed to produce organized collagen to improve the appearance of a depressed scar. Often, multiple treatments are done at monthly intervals and provide the best smoothing effect. There is no laser technique that will completely eliminate a scar at this time.

Additional Health Tips to Enhance Healing:

▸ Prevention is the best medicine. Skin conditions should be addressed before scarring occurs. In his practice, Dr. Braun notes that if acne, for instance, is not resolved within six months, scars form in 90 percent of cases. If you have skin problems, seek treatment as soon as possible.

▸ Never pick or scratch a scab. Pulling at the skin damages the dermis and ultimately leads to scarring.

▸ Topical creams containing sulforaphane can aid with scar reduction.

▸ Apply GLA Skin Oil at bedtime.

▸ Rose hip oil, also known as rosa mosqueta oil, can be used to help moisturize the skin and reduce the appearance of scar tissue. Do not apply it to an open wound. Apply twice daily for two to three months for improvement. The oil's high content of EFAs provide topical moisture to the skin and relieve inflammation.

SKIN TAGS

A skin tag is a fleshy, small, raised growth that is darker in color and is often found on the neck, upper and lower eyelids, in the groin area, and under the arms. These are typical places where rubbing and/or wear and tear occur. Although there is a genetic component to skin tags, lifestyle is another factor. Skin tags also occur during pregnancy due to increased growth and hormonal fluctuations.

Skin tags are strongly associated with prediabetes (lso called insulin resistance) and type-2 diabetes. In those with insulin resistance, insulin becomes ineffective at pushing sugar into the cells and consequently, the blood sugar builds up and the body keeps producing more insulin in an attempt to normalize blood sugar. Eventually, the pancreas becomes exhausted and diabetes results. We have an epidemic of type-2 diabetes and early detection can prevent the development of this deadly disease. Diabetics, on average, live 10 to 15 years less than non-diabetics. Dozens of studies show that as few as three skin tags on the body are linked to an increased risk of diabetes. Research has also shown that those with skin tags have higher cholesterol, triglycerides (blood fats), blood sugar, and C-reactive protein (CRP) than those without skin tags; these features are all risk factors for diabetes and cardiovascular disease. Those people with elevated CRP, a marker for inflammation in the body, are four times more likely to develop diabetes. So although skin tags look bad, they are actually a warning sign for diabetes that we should not ignore.

PRESCRIPTION FOR HEALTH

Nutrient	Dosage	Action
Glucosmart	1-2 capsules daily. Each capsule contains: D-chiro-inositol (Chirositol™) 600 mg Chromium picolinate 2.2 mcg	Normalizes blood sugar and insulin; reduces appetite and improves serotonin. Skin tags fall off when blood sugar normalizes.

Nutrient	Dosage	Action
Multivitamin with minerals (contains no iron); Multismart	As directed; should contain the following nutrients: Vitamin A 1250 IU	Promotes smooth, clear skin
	Beta carotene 7500 IU Folic acid 500 mcg P-5-P (vitamin B6) 30 mg	Facilitates the breakdown of excess hormones
	Vitamin B3 15 mg, along with other B vitamins Vitamin D 500 IU	Promotes healing of the skin
	Vitamin E 100 IU	Acts as an antioxidant and encourages tissue repair
	Zinc 7.5 mg	Essential for healthy immune function
	Chromium polynicotinate 100 mcg	Improves glucose tolerance and fatty acid metabolism
	Selenomethionine 50 mcg	To enhance glutathione and fight bacteria
GLA Skin Oil	Adults: 4-6 tsp per day Children: 1-2 tsp daily Each tsp contains GLA 500 mg	Reduces inflammation in the skin; improves moisture retention
Cala-Q Plus	2 softgels daily	Anti-inflammatory; helps prevent against insulin resistance; cuts diabetes and heart disease risk
CLA Plus with Green Tea Extract	6 softgels daily. Each softgel contains: Conjugated linoleic acid (CLA from safflower oil) 730 mg Camellia sinensis (Green tea extract) 113.3 mg	Being obese or overweight exacerbates skin tags. CLA Plus speeds up metabolism, reduces inflammation, and offers anti-inflammatory and anti-cancer benefits.
Estrosmart	2-4 capsules daily. Each 2 capsules contain: Indole-3-carbinol 150 mg Sulforaphane 200 mcg D-glucarate 150 mg Curcumin 50 mg Rosemary 25 mg	Balances hormones; detoxifies excess estrogens; prevents estrogens from converting into cancer-causing estrogens. Contains the equivalent cancer-

Nutrient	Dosage	Action
	DIM 50 mg Green tea extract 100 mg	protecting plant nutrients as 1 kg of cruciferous vegetables.

General Considerations/Options by Dr. Braun:

Skin tags are often unsightly, especially around the eyelids and sides of the neck. These lesions are easy to excise.

Additional Health Tips to Enhance Healing:

▸ Do not pluck, tweeze or otherwise attempt to remove skin tags by yourself because you may cause an infection. In skin tags, all the layers of the skin have been squished up, producing a darker color, and they usually contain a blood vessel. That is why they bleed more than expected when irritated.

▸ Obesity can make skin tags worse. Maintaining a healthy weight is essential to your health. Glucosmart and CLA Plus are clinically tested formulas for weight loss. Few supplements pass Health Canada's stringent regulatory requirements for weight loss claims. Both Glucosmart and CLA Plus have been approved by Health Canada.

▸ Besides skin tags, if you have excess belly fat, acne, male-pattern facial hair growth (e.g. above the lip and on the chin), skin tags, diabetes and pre-diabetes, these are classic symptoms of elevated insulin and male hormones. Estrosmart and Glucosmart are the best combination for combating insulin resistance, rebalancing hormones, losing weight and reducing belly fat.

STRETCH MARKS

Stretch marks are actually a kind of scar that is caused when the skin is pulled and thinned to the point that collagen and elastin lose their integrity and cannot return to normal. These whitish, wriggly-looking marks tend to appear around the hips, belly, and on the insides of the knees and outsides of the breasts. Pregnant women, adolescents and people who gain weight often develop stretch marks.

PRESCRIPTION FOR HEALTH

Nutrient	Dosage	Action
Collagen Plus	10 drops daily in juice; each drop contains: Silicic acid 1 mg Biotin 50 mcg	Important for building and retaining a healthy skin matrix. Silicic acid and biotin help build collagen.
GLA Skin Oil	Adults: 4-6 tsp per day; children; 1-2 tsp daily Each tsp contains 500 mg of GLA	Reduces inflammation in the skin; improves moisture retention
Sulforaphane	Apply topically	Repairs skin damage; restores and maintains skin integrity

General Considerations/Options by Dr. Braun:
Thin, white scars are one of the most difficult cosmetic conditions to treat. One can obtain a 30 to 50 percent improvement with radiofrequency tissue heating using devices such as Thermage® or Accent® RF. This modality is often combined with fractional resurfacing, making tiny perforations in the skin resulting in new collagen formation by the body's natural healing processes.

Additional Health Tips to Enhance Healing:
▸ During pregnancy, many women swear by anti-stretch oils, lotions and creams that contain moisturizing ingredients such as vitamin E, rose hip oil, cocoa butter, shea butter, avocado butter or olive oil.
▸ Rapid weight loss and gain are the biggest contributors to stretch marks. If your weight is fluctuating, consult a naturopathic doctor or a qualified health professional to guide you in weight maintenance decisions.

UNWANTED HAIR
It is not uncommon for women to grow too much hair or to have male pattern hair growth. Typical areas include above the upper lip, whiskers on the chin, and darker, coarser hairs on the belly. Hair growth starts in puberty and speeds during pregnancy. Hairs tend to darken and thicken with age. While ethnicity somewhat determines hair growth, another common underlying reason is hormone imbalance. Unwanted hair growth can be due to higher

levels of testosterone. It can be a symptom of polycystic ovarian syndrome (PCOS), a disorder where male hormones are excessively high and there may be many fluid-filled cysts present. In this disorder, excess hormones increase the production of male hormones that cause acne and coarse hair growth. PCOS is also associated with the production of too much insulin (hyperinsulinemia) and impaired glucose metabolism. In menopausal and postmenopausal women, however, unwanted hair growth is most often due to high levels of prolactin and low levels of estrogen.

PRESCRIPTION FOR HEALTH

Nutrient	Dosage	Action
Multivitamin with minerals (contains no iron); Multismart	As directed; should contain the following nutrients: Vitamin A 1250 IU Beta carotene 7500 IU Folic acid 500 mcg P-5-P (vitamin B6) 30 mg	Facilitates the breakdown of excess hormones
	Vitamin B3 15 mg, along with other B vitamins Vitamin D 500 IU Vitamin E 100 IU	Acts as an antioxidant and encourages tissue repair
	Zinc 7.5 mg	Essential for healthy immune function
	Chromium polynicotinate 100 mcg	Improves glucose tolerance and fatty acid metabolism
Glucosmart	1-2 capsules daily. Each capsule contains: D-chiro-inositol (Chirositol™) 600 mg Chromium picolinate 2.2 mcg	Normalizes blood sugar and insulin; reduces male hormones in women; excellent for PCOS, traditionally a difficult condition to treat.
Estrosmart	2-4 capsules daily. Each 2 capsules contain: Indole-3-carbinol 150 mg Sulforaphane 200 mcg D-glucarate 150 mg Curcumin 50 mg Rosemary 25 mg DIM 50 mg Green tea extract 100 mg	Balances hormones; detoxifies excess estrogens and prevents good estrogens from converting into cancer-causing estrogens.

Nutrient	Dosage	Action
GLA Skin Oil	2 to 6 tsp of GLA per day	Promotes hormone balance and a healthy inflammation response to reduce stress

General Considerations/Options by Dr. Braun:

In 1996, Dr. Braun was one of six physicians in the world who were performing laser hair removal. Now one can find a laser hair removal clinic on virtually every corner in the Western hemisphere, and laser hair removal has become the most popular laser procedure in North America. However, not all laser devices (and clinics) are created equally. A patient should choose a clinic with a good reputation and with many years of experience. There are many clinics that "guarantee" laser hair removal results. It is impossible to guarantee a hair-free state for life. There is no such thing; the name laser hair removal is a misnomer. It should be called laser hair reduction, as the laser reduces the density and caliber of the hair shaft. The laser, however, does not remove the hair shaft. Once the hair follicle is miniaturized, the area appears to have less hair. A good hair removal clinic will have a medical director who is available to deal with any potential complications. Multiple treatments will be necessary for hair reduction, and some people will be resistant to the laser; for example, patients with polycystic ovarian syndrome.

Additional Health Tips to Enhance Healing:

▶ Focus on a diet rich in vegetables providing at least 25 g of fiber daily to help naturally eliminate excess testosterone via the bowels. Avoid foods that might aggravate the condition such as conventional meat and dairy products.

▶ Maintaining a healthy weight is essential for hormone balance, particularly in women who are dealing with PCOS. If you are overweight, read Lorna's book, *A Smart Woman's Guide to Weight Loss.*

▶ Apply topical estriol, which reduces the amount of testosterone/male hormones in the skin, thereby stopping male facial hair growth. See page 61 for the prescription for estriol and more information.

▶ Apply topical GLA Skin Oil to areas of the face. GLA has been shown to normalize testosterone in the skin and also hair follicles.

▶ There are plenty of at-home products for short-term hair removal such as waxes, depilatory creams, tweezers and razors.

VARICOSE/SPIDER VEINS

Visible veins affect 80 percent of women. Spider veins are those small red, blue and purple blood vessels that appear most frequently on the face and thighs. Varicose veins are larger in diameter and may appear raised with a bluish color. The leading causes of spider and varicose veins are heredity, aging, pregnancy and hormonal changes. Varicose veins can also be related to more serious vein disorders so they require a careful evaluation prior to treatment. Effective non-surgical treatments for both varicose and spider veins are available.

PRESCRIPTION FOR HEALTH

Nutrient	Dosage	Action
Multivitamin with minerals (contains no iron); Multismart	As directed; should contain the following nutrients: Vitamin A 1250 IU Beta carotene 7500 IU Folic acid 500 mcg P-5-P (vitamin B6) 30 mg Vitamin B3 15 mg, along with other B vitamins Vitamin D 500 IU Vitamin E 100 IU Zinc 7.5 mg Chromium polynicotinate 100 mg Selenomethionine 50 mcg	Supports immune function; potent antioxidant; supports vein integrity; detoxifies the liver; prevents deficiency; repairs blood vessel walls; prevents blood clotting and bruising; improves circulation.
Veinsmart	3 capsules per day with food, containing: Diosmin (micronized) 900 mg Horse Chestnut Seed Extract 500 mg Butcher's Broom Extract 100 mg Hesperidin 100 mg	Supports vein health and reduces varicose veins; eliminates hemorrhoids; eliminates heavy feeling legs and swelling in the legs
Collagen Plus	Mix 10 drops daily in juice. Each drop contains: Silicic acid 1 mg Biotin 50 mcg	Found to enhance artery and vein health
Ground flax seed (high lignans)	1 to 2 tablespoons daily	Soothes intestinal lining and promotes elimination

Nutrient	Dosage	Action
Cala-Q Plus	2 softgels daily containing: 1000 mg calamari oil providing 720 mg of DHA and 280 mg of EPA	Helps heal skin
Bromelain	500-1000 mg after every meal	Anti-inflammatory, shown to prevent hard, lumpy skin around bulging varicose veins
Blueberry, Cranberry Mangosteen, Pomegranate	500 mg per day	Improves the integrity of capillaries, veins and protects collagen from damage in varicose veins. Potent antioxidant effect.

General Considerations/Options by Dr. Braun:

Ultrasound has revolutionized the treatment of varicose veins. The proper method to treat varicose veins in the twenty-first century is to perform an ultrasonic map of all the veins in your lower limbs. This takes about 40 minutes and is completely painless and non-invasive. Following the mapping procedure, the doctor can see the precise location of the failed venous valves. All varicose vein disease is due to failed venous valves. The valves are present to prevent blood from falling down to your toes. The venous blood is supposed to go against gravity back to the heart, but if the valves have failed, the blood falls and the vein starts to dilate. Using an ultrasound, a phlebologist can inject foam into a vein causing it to collapse permanently. Surgically stripping veins is no longer necessary. Surgically stripping veins is not recommended because it results in unsightly scars and can lead to further vein growth. A laser can also be used with excellent results. With proper follow up, successful resolution of vein disease exceeds 90 percent. A patient can check for a vein specialist through the American Board of Phlebology.

Additional Health Tips to Enhance Healing:

▶ Reduce your weight; even 10 extra pounds puts added pressure on your venous system.

▶ Eat plenty of vegetables to ensure adequate fiber intake to improve bowel movements.

▸ Drink at least 8 to 10 glasses of pure, filtered water every day. Water maintains a healthy level of blood volume and prevents constipation.

▸ Apply witch hazel ointment topically twice a day to reduce swelling and tone veins.

▸ Avoid standing or sitting for long periods. Regular exercise is mandatory for circulation disorders and maintaining weight.

▸ Stop smoking. Nicotine constricts blood vessels.

▸ When traveling for long periods, make sure that you stand up and move around every 20 minutes to keep circulation going and prevent blood clots.

▸ Supportive elastic stockings for varicose veins in combination with the above recommendations can dramatically reduce the appearance of unsightly veins. However, you should be properly measured and fitted for compression stockings. The latest vein compression stockings are very attractive and can easily be worn every day.

▸ Hydrotherapy can alleviate pain and improve circulation. Fill a bathtub full of cold water, get in and walk on the spot for 20 minutes (Use an anti-slip tub mat.) An alternative is to spray cold water on the legs, front and back, for ten seconds every morning in the shower.

▸ When sitting or lying down, raise the legs above the heart for 20 minutes every day.

▸ Shift your weight and stand on your toes periodically if you must stand for long periods of time. If you sit at a desk, wiggle your toes and flex your legs to promote blood flow. Do not cross your legs.

▸ Do not scratch veins if they are itchy because you may cause further damage.

WARTS

Warts are a viral skin infection caused by any one of the almost 60 strains of the human papilloma virus (HPV) and they affect a large percentage of the population. Plantar warts are located on the soles of the feet and are difficult to eliminate. Warts commonly appear on the hands, feet, nails and face, but can appear anywhere on the body.

A healthy immune system can help to fight off the HPV virus most of the time. The recurrence of warts suggests that the immune system is suppressed or weakened.

PRESCRIPTION FOR HEALTH

Nutrient	Dosage	Action
Multivitamin with minerals (contains no iron); Multismart	As directed; should contain the following nutrients: Vitamin A 1250 IU Beta carotene 7500 IU Folic acid 500 mcg P-5-P (vitamin B6) 30 mg Vitamin B3 15 mg, along with other B vitamins Vitamin D 500 IU Vitamin E 100 IU Zinc 7.5 mg Chromium polynicotinate 100 mcg Selenomethionine 50 mcg	Promotes smooth, clear skin Facilitates the breakdown of excess hormones Promotes healing of the skin Acts as an antioxidant and encourages tissue repair Essential for healthy immune function Improves glucose tolerance and fatty acid metabolism To enhance glutathione and fight bacteria
Immunosmart	Two capsules daily.	Regulates immune function, enhances virus-fighting activity, controls cortisol, and enhances immune activity.
Probiotic Plus	2 capsules daily. Each capsule contains: 2.5 billion active cells of BB536 Bifidobacterium 250 mg of whole cranberry extract	Enhances immune function and intestinal flora and aids digestion
Oil of oregano	3-5 drops twice daily in water or juice and applied topically to the wart	Antiviral; antibacterial
Garlic	Two capsules daily and plenty of fresh garlic in foods	Boosts immunity; helps fight viruses
Wobenzym® homeopathic remedy	3-5 tablets daily	Disables viruses

General Considerations/Options by Dr. Braun

An old-fashioned treatment that may work for you is to cover the wart with duct tape. Try this every day for a month to determine if the wart will regress.

Additional Health Tips to Enhance Healing:

▸ Buff the wart with an emory board and then place a piece of duct tape on the wart. Leave it on and the wart will disappear. Reapply if needed.

▸ Quite often, common and plantar warts will resolve themselves without treatment. Do not try to remove warts by yourself.

> **HPV Virus, Cervical Dysplasia and Cancer**
>
> Warts are contagious and can be transmitted sexually. When they appear on the cervix, it is critical that they be treated aggressively because some strains of HPV are the main cause of cervical dysplasia, a precancerous condition. PAP smears save lives by discovering abnormal cells early enough to prevent death from cervical cancer. Every adult woman from the age of 18 should have an annual PAP test to ensure her cervix is health. But what can be done when the test comes back abnormal?
>
> As we mentioned in Chapter 4, the nutrient indole-3-carbinol (I3C) can reverse abnormal cervical lesions before they can develop into cancer. In one study, 30 women with advanced cervical lesions took 200-400 mg of I3C daily. Fifty percent in the treatment group had complete regression of their lesions. No one in the placebo group had complete regression of their lesions. Indole-3-carbinol is found in Estrosmart in the dosages used in the study to reverse abnormal cells. Estrosmart also contains other nutrients, including calcium D-glucarate, diindolylmethane, rosemary, sulforaphane, tumeric and green tea—all researched to help prevent female cancers and to keep estrogens from converting to cancer-causing estrogens. With Estrosmart, you find that abnormal PAP tests to will return to normal.

WRINKLES

As you have hopefully learned by now, your skin is more than an inactive barrier between you and the external world. Your skin is alive—a reflection of internal and external processes such as those that we have detailed earlier in this book. Diet, habits, topical agents, and age-management technologies can all help slow the ticking of time.

PRESCRIPTION FOR HEALTH

Nutrient	Dosage	Action
Multivitamin with minerals (contains no iron); Multismart	As directed; should contain the following nutrients: Vitamin A 1250 IU	Promotes smooth, clear skin
	Beta carotene 7500 IU Folic acid 500 mcg P-5-P (vitamin B6) 30 mg Vitamin B3 15 mg, along with other B vitamins Vitamin D 500 IU	Promotes healing of the skin
	Vitamin E 100 IU	Acts as an antioxidant and encourages tissue repair
	Zinc 7.5 mg	Essential for healthy immune function
	Chromium polynicotinate 100 mcg Selenomethionine 50 mcg	Improves glucose tolerance and fatty acid metabolism To enhance glutathione and fight bacteria
Collagen Plus	Mix 10 drops daily in juice. Each drop contains: Silicic acid 1 mg Biotin 50 mcg	Important for building and retaining a healthy skin matrix. Silicic acid and biotin help build collagen.
Active Collagen	2000 mg per day with food	Decreases lines and wrinkles; enhances skin moisture
GLA Skin Oil	2-6 tsp per day. Each tsp contains GLA 500 mg.	Reduces inflammation in the skin; improves moisture retention
Cala-Q Plus with coenzyme Q10	2 softgels daily	Helps heal the skin. Important to prevent free radical damage; improves skin structure.
French Maritime Pine Bark Extract	As directed	Protects against free radical damage, reduces wrinkles, enhances hydration and elasticity, improves micro-circulation

General Considerations/Options by Dr. Braun:

Wrinkles can basically be classified as fine lines on the face or deeper grooves. Both can be improved by supporting the underlying skin with a filler. I use only biodegradable fillers that are natural to the skin structure, like hyaluronic acid (HA). Go to page 63 for in-depth information on hyaluronic acid fillers such as Juvéderm® and Restylane®.

The reason an infant's skin feels so plump and smooth is due to the hyaluronic acid under their skin. It has been estimated that our face loses about one to two percent of its hyaluronic acid content annually after age 20. In addition, if a person has a healthy body weight due to proper exercise and diet, they will also lose subcutaneous fat from their face, especially after age 35 to 40. The loss of HA and fat under the facial skin results in deep grooves, and ultimately gravity takes this loose skin downwards and we see sagging. In the past, this was addressed with a face lift.

Multiple studies have now shown that the restoration of HA under the skin will plump out those deep grooves and fine lines, resulting in skin lifting and smoother skin. This can be accomplished with HA filler injections or fat transfer. It is completely safe and results in a very natural appearance as no skin is cut or pulled. Unfortunately, the concept of volume loss as the hallmark of the aging face is not understood by the vast majority of people. Another advantage of HA is that if you do not like it, it can be dissolved within a day using another natural enzyme called hyaluronidase.

Having an eraser available makes HA particularly attractive as a filler. HA can be used anywhere on the face—for the hollow eyes, tear troughs, mid-face collapse, etc. The mid-face area is especially important to keep up as a loss of mid-face cheek fat results in a deep groove and a lack of support because the tear trough under the eye allows the eye bag to expand. This process results in a tired look, and once the eye bags are severely herniated outwards, only surgery can alleviate the look by removing and repositioning the fat. Anterior mid-face projections are also a hallmark of a youthful face.

Additional Health Tips to Enhance Healing:

▸ Use Celadrin Super Rich Skin Therapy Cream daily for smooth, soft skin. Celadrin has been researched for its ability to reduce pain and inflammation as well as improve the appearance of wrinkles. In a study at the University of California, Celadrin (10 percent) cream was applied twice daily for 21 days. A dramatic reduction in skin wrinkles and enhanced hydration and elasticity was noted in the 28 women taking part in this trial.

Celadrin Super Rich Skin Therapy Cream also contains hylauronic acid and chamomile extract for added skin-smoothing properties.

▶ Incorporate plenty of vegetables and spices into your diet. Plant-based foods contain polyphenols, which are naturally occurring compounds with skin-protective properties. Polyphenols can be found in onions (flavonols), cacao beans, grape seeds (proanthocyanidins), tea (catechins), apples and red wine (flavonols and catechins), citrus fruits (flavanones), and berries and cherries (anthocyanidins). Because the body utilizes this type of anti-oxidant rapidly, it is important to replenish your internal stores with daily consumption.

▶ Curcumin, resveratrol, coenzyme Q10 and carotenoids have also all been found to offer skin-protective benefits.

▶ Everyone should consider applying a quality vitamin A (retinol) product to their skin. Retinol inhibits collagen destruction, and since it is stored by the liver, it is not possible to simply eat more vitamin A in order to achieve higher levels of retinol in the skin. One has to apply it topically. Retinol can be irritating, so one should start slowly every second to third night and increase the frequency of application as tolerated. The concentration should be in the range of 0.05 to 1 percent. Most people will not tolerate retinol with a 1 percent concentration more than one to two times per week.

ABOUT THE AUTHORS

Dr. Martin Braun is one of the most accomplished and respected cosmetic rejuvenation physicians practicing in the Vancouver area. His goal is to help everyone achieve beautiful skin for life, beginning at any age. After receiving his M.D. from the University of British Columbia (UBC) in 1984, Dr. Braun completed his core surgical training at Vancouver General Hospital. As a pioneer in laser medicine, Dr. Braun has the distinction of being the first doctor in Canada to perform laser hair removal over 15 years ago. He currently injects more Botox® than any other practitioner in Canada! He is the Medical Director of Vancouver Laser and Skin Care Centre Inc.

Lorna Vanderhaeghe is Canada's leading women's natural health expert. She has been researching nutritional medicine for over 30 years. With degrees in biochemistry and nutrition, she is the author of twelve books including *A Smart Woman's Guide to Hormones* and *A Smart Woman's Guide to Weight Loss*. In 2009, Lorna won the Canadian Health Food Association's most prestigious award, the Hall of Fame Award. In 2013, Lorna was listed as one of Canada's top one hundred female entrepreneurs. She has a free monthly newsletter and her website is www.hormonehelp.com.

REFERENCES

A

Altemus M, et al. Stress-induced changes in skin barrier function in healthy women. J Invest Dermatol. 2001;117(2):309-17.

Andreassi M, et al. Efficacy of gamma linolenic acid in the treatment of patients with atopic dermatitis. J Int Med Res. 1997;25:266-74.

Antoniou C, et al. Photoaging: prevention and topical treatments. Am J Clin Dermatol. 2010;11(2):95-102.

Ascher B, et al. Efficacy and safety of botulinum toxin type A in the treatment of lateral crow's feet: double-blind, placebo-controlled, dose-ranging study. Dermatol Surg. 2009;35(10):1478-86.

Auborn KJ, et al. Lifespan is prolonged in autoimmune-prone (NZB/NZW) F1 mice fed a diet supplemented with indole-3-carbinol. J Nutr. 2003;133:3610-3.

B

Bae JY, et al. Dietary compound ellagic acid alleviates skin wrinkle and inflammation induced by UV-B irradiation. Exp Dermatol. 2010;19(8):e182-90.

Barcelo S, et al. CYP2E1—mediated mechanism of anti-genotoxicity of the broccoli constituent sulforaphane. Carcinogenesis. 1996;17:277-82.

Beitner H. Randomized, placebo controlled, double blind study on the clinical efficacy of a cream containing 5% alpha lipoic acid related to photoageing of facial skin. Br J Dermatol. 2003;149(4):841-9.

Belcaro G, et al. Venous ulcers: microcirculatory improvement and faster healing with local use of Pycnogenol. Angiology. 2005;56(6):699-705.

Bernhard MK, et al. Botulinum toxin injections for chronic migraine in adolescents: An early therapeutic option in the transition from neuropaediatrics to neurology. Fortschr Neurol Psychiatr. 2014;82(1):39-42.

Blazsó G, et al. Pycnogenol accelerates wound healing and reduces scar formation. Phytother Res. 2004;18(7):579-581.

Boelsma E, et al. Human skin condition and its associations with nutrient concentrations in serum and diet. Am J Clin Nutr. 2003;77(2):348-55.

Bosche T and D Platt. Effect of borage oil consumption on fatty acid metabolism, transepidermal water loss and skin parameters in elderly people. Arch Gerontol Geriatr. 2001;30:139-150.

Brignall MS. Prevention and treatment of cancer with indole-3-carbinol. Altern Med Rev. 2001;6(6):580-9.

Bruce S. Cosmeceuticals for the attenuation of extrinsic and intrinsic dermal aging. J Drugs Dermatol. 2008;7(2Suppl):s17-22.

Burke KE, et al. Synergistic damage by UVA radiation and pollutants. Toxicol Ind Health. 2009;25(4-5):219-24.

Businco L, et al. Breast milk from mothers of children with newly developed atopic eczema has low levels of chain polyunsaturated fatty acids. J Allergy Clin Immunol. 1993;91:1134.

C

Carruthers JA, et al. A multicenter, double-blind, randomized, placebo-controlled study of the efficacy and safety of botulinum toxin type A in the treatment of glabellar lines. J Am Acad Dermatol. 2002;46(6):840-9.

Chalk CH, et al. Medical treatment for botulism. Cochrane Database Syst Rev. 2011;16(3):CD008123.

Chen DZ, et al. Indole-3-carbinol and diindolylmethane induce apoptosis of human cervical cancer cells and in murine HPV16-transgenic preneoplastic cervical epithelium. J Nutr. 2001;131(12):3294-302.

Chen S. Clinical uses of botulinum neurotoxins: current indications, limitations and future developments. Toxins. 2012;4(10):913-39.

Chida M, et al. In vitro testing of antioxidants and biochemical end-point in bovine retinal tissue. Ophthalmic Res. 1999;31(6):407-15.

Chiu A, et al. The response of skin disease to stress: changes in the severity of acne vulgaris as affected by examination stress. Arch Dermatol. 2003;139(7):897-900.

Clapper ML, et al. Preclinical clinical evaluation of broccoli supplements as inducers of glutathione and S-transferase activity. Clin Cancer Res. 1997;3:25-30.

Cornblatt BS, et al. Preclinical and clinical evaluation of sulforaphane for chemoprevention in the breast. Carcinogenesis. 2007;28(7):1485-1490.

Cosgrove MC, et al. Dietary nutrient intakes and skin-aging appearance among middle-aged American women. Am J Clin Nutr. 2007;86(4):1225-1231.

Cover CM, et al. Indole-3-carbinol and tamoxifen cooperate to arrest the cell cycle of MCF-7 human breast cancer cells. Cancer Res. 1999;59(6):1244-51.

Devaraj S, et al. Supplementation with a pine bark extract rich in polyphenols increases plasma antioxidant capacity and alters the plasma lipoprotein profile. Lipids. 2002;37(10):931-4.

D

Dinkova-Kostova AT, et al. Protection against UV-light-induced skin carcinogenesis in SKH-1 high-risk mice by sulforaphane-containing broccoli sprout extracts. Cancer Lett. 2006;240(2):243-52.

Downing, et al. Essential fatty acids and acne. J Am Acad Dermatol. 1986;14:221-5.

Dreher F, et al. Topical melatonin in combination with vitamins E and C protects skin from ultraviolet-induced erythema: a human study in vivo. Br J Dermatol. 1999;139(2): 332-9.

F

Fahey JW, et al. Antioxidant functions of sulforaphane: a potent inducer of Phase II detoxication enzymes. Food Chem Toxicol. 1999;37:973-9.

Fahey JW, et al. Broccoli sprouts: an exceptionally rich source of inducers of enzymes that protect against chemical carcinogens. Proc Natl Acad Sci. 1997;94:10367-72.

Fahey JW, et al. Sulforaphane inhibits extracellular, intracellular, and antibiotic-resistant strains of Helicobacter pylori and prevents benzo[a]pyrene-induced stomach tumors. Proc Natl Acad Sci. 2002;99:7610-7615.

Fisher GJ, et al. Collagen fragmentation promotes oxidative stress and elevates matrix metalloproteinase-1 in fibroblasts in aged human skin. Am J Pathol. 2009;174(1):101-14.

Fitzpatrick DF, et al. Endothelium-dependent vascular effects of Pycnogenol. J Cardiovasc Pharmacol. 1998;329(4):509-515.

Frydoonfar HR, et al. Sulforaphane inhibits growth of a colon cancer cell line. Colorectal Dis. 2004;6(1):28-31.

Frydoonfar HR, et al. The effect of indole-3-carbinol and sulforaphane on a prostate cancer cell line. ANZ J Surg. 2003;73(3):154-6.

Fuller B, et al. Anti-inflammatory effects of CoQ10 and colorless carotenoids. J Cosmet Dermatol. 2006;5(1):30-8.

G

Gao X, et al. Endocrine disruption by indole-3-carbinol and tamoxifen: blockage of ovulation. Toxicol Appl Pharmacol. 2002;183(3):179-88.

Gingras D, et al. Induction of medulloblastoma cell apoptosis by sulforaphane, a dietary anticarcinogen from Brassica vegetables. Cancer Lett. 2004;203(1):35-43.

Grimm T, et al. Antioxidant activity and inhibition of matrix-metalloproteinases by metabolites of maritime pine bark extract (Pycnogenol). Free Radic Biol Med. 2004;36(6):811-822.

Grimm T, et al. Inhibition of NF-kB activation and MMP-9 secretion by plasma of human volunteers after ingestion of maritime pine bark extract (Pycnogenol). J Inflamm. 2006;3(1):1-15.

Guinot C, et al. Effect of hormonal replacement therapy on skin biophysical properties of menopausal women. Skin Res Technol. 2005;11(3):201-4.

H

Haftek M, et al. Clinical, biometric and structural evaluation of the long-term effects of a topical treatment with ascorbic acid and madecassoside in photodamaged human skin. Exp Dermatol. 2008;17(11):946-52.

Hall G, et al. Estrogen and skin: the effects of estrogen, menopause, and hormone replacement therapy on the skin. J Am Acad Dermatol. 2005:53(4):569-72.

Hansen TM, et al. treatment of rheumatoid arthritis with prostaglandin E1 precursors cis-linoleic acid and gamma-linolenic acid. Sacnd J Rheumatol. 1983;12(2):85-8.

Haristoy X, et al. Efficacy of sulforaphane in eradicating Helicobacter pylori in human gastric xenografts implanted in nude mice. Antimicrob Agents Chemother. 2003;47(12): 3982-3984.

Hecht SS. Chemoprevention of cancer by isothiocyanates, modifiers of carcinogen metabolism. J Nutr. 1999;129:768S-774S. Review.

Henz, BM. Double-blind, multicentre analysis of the efficacy of borage oil in patients with atopic eczema. Br J Dermatol. 1999;140:685-88.

Hoppe U, et al. Coenzyme Q10, a cutaneous antioxidant and energizer. Biofactors. 1999;9(2-4):371-8.

Horrobin DF. Essential fatty acid metabolism and its modification in atopic eczema. A J Clinc Nutr. 2000;71(suppl):367S-372S.

Humbert P, et al. Topical vitamin C in the treatment of photoaged skin. Clinical, topographical and ultrastructural evaluation: double-blind study vs. placebo. Eur J Dermatol. 2003;12(3):237-44.

J

Jackson SJ, et al. Sulforaphane: a naturally occurring mammary carcinoma mitotic inhibitor which disrupts tubulin polymerization. Carcinogenesis. 2003;25(2):219-27.

Jang M, et al. Cancer chemopreventive activity of resveratrol, a natural product derived from grapes. Science. 1997;275(5297):218-20.

K

Kall MA, et al. Effects of dietary broccoli on human drug metabolising activity. Cancer Lett. 1997;114:169-70.

Kawamura A, et al. Dietary supplementation of gamma-linolenic acid improves skin parameters in subjects with dry skin and mild atopic dermatitis. J Oleo Sci. 2011;60(12): 597-607.

Kelloff GJ, et al. Progress in cancer chemoprevention: development of diet-derived chemopreventive agents. J Nutr. 2000;130:467S-471S.

Kerns ML, et al. Reprogramming of keratin biosynthesis by sulforaphane restores skin integrity in epidermolysis bullosa simplex. Proc Natl Acad Sci. 2007;104(36):14460-5.

Kiecolt-Glaser JK, et al. Slowing of wound healing by psychological stress. Lancet. 1995;346(8984):1194-6.

Kim BR, et al. Effects of glutathione on antioxidant response element-mediated gene expression and apoptosis elicited by sulforaphane. Cancer Res. 2003;63(21):7520-5.

Knuutinen A, et al. Smoking affects collagen synthesis and extracellular matrix turnover in human skin. Br J Dermatol. 2002;146(4):588-94.

Kolm RH, et al. Isothiocyanates as substrates for human glutathione transferases: structure-activity studies. Biochem J. 1995;311:453-9.

L

Lima CF, et al. Curcumin induces heme oxygenase-1 in normal human skin fibroblasts through redox signaling: relevance for anti-aging intervention. Mol Nutr Food Res. 2011;55(3):430-42.

M

Mac-Mary S, et al. Could a photobiological test be a suitable method to assess the anti-oxidant effect of a nutritional supplement (Glisodin)? Eur J Dermatol. 2007;17(3):54-5.

Maheo K, et al. Inhibition of cytochromes P-450 and induction of glutathione S- transferases by sulforaphane in primary human and rat hepatocytes. Cancer Res. 1997;57:3649-52.

Marini A, et al. Pycnogenol® effects on skin elasticity and hydration coincide with increased gene expressions of collagen type I and hyaluronic acid synthase in women. Skin Pharmacol Physiol. 2012;25(2):86-92.

Masaki H. Role of antioxidants in the skin: anti-aging effects. J Dermatol Sci. 2010;58(2):85-90.

Mayo Clinic. Sun damage. 2014. Retrieved from http://www.mayoclinic.org/sun-damage/sls-20076973

McAlindon TE, et al. Indole-3-carbinol in women with SLE: effect on estrogen metabolism and disease activity. Lupus. 2001; 10(11):779-83.

Melnick BC. Evidence for acne-promoting effects of milk and other insulinotropic dairy products. Nestle Nutr Workshop Ser Pediatr Program. 2011;67:131-45.

Muta-Takada K, et al. Coenzyme Q10 protects against oxidative stress-induced cell death and enhances the synthesis of basement membrane components in dermal and epidermal cells. Biofactors. 2009;35(5):435-41.

N

Nachshon-Kedmi M, et al. Indole-3-carbinol and 3,3'-diindolylmethane induce apoptosis in human prostate cancer cells. Food Chem Toxicol. 2003;41(6):745-52.

Namjoshi S, et al. Cyclic peptides as potential therapeutic agents for skin disorders. Biopolymers. 2010;94(5):673-80.

Namjoshi S, et al. Skin peptides: biological activity and therapeutic opportunities. J Pharma Sci. 2008;97(7):2524-42.

Nestle M. Broccoli sprouts as inducers of carcinogen-detoxifying enzyme systems: clinical, dietary, and policy implications. Proc Natl Acad Sci. 1997;94:11149-51. Review.

Nestle M. Broccoli sprouts in cancer prevention. Nutr Rev. 1998;56:127-30. Review.

Nichols JA, et al. Skin photoprotection by natural polyphenols: anti-inflammatory, antioxidant and DNA repair mechanisms. Arch Dermatol Res. 2010;302(2):71-83.

Nijhoff WA, et al. Effects of consumption of Brussels sprouts on plasma and urinary glutathione S-transferase class-alpha and -pi in humans. Carcinogenesis. 1995;16:955-7.

Nissen HP, et al. The effect of gamma linolenic acid on skin smoothness, humidity and TEWL – A clinical study. Inform. 1995;6(4):5-19.

Nutra Ingredients. Fruit extracts offer hope in skin cancer prevention. Oct. 2003. www.nutraingredients.com/Research/Fruit-extracts-offer-hope-in-skin-cancer-prevention

O

Orengo IF. Influence of dietary menhaden oil upon carcinogenesis and various cutaneous responses to ultraviolet radiation. Photochem Photobiol. 1989;49(1):71-77.

Osborne MP. Chemoprevention of breast cancer. Surg Clin North Am. 1999;79(5):1207-21.

P

Pageon H, et al. Reconstructed skin modified by glycation of the dermal equivalent as a model for skin aging and its potential use to evaluate anti-glycation molecules. Exp Gerontol. 2008;43(6):584-8.

Pascucci B, et al. Role of nucleotide excision repair proteins in oxidative DNA damage repair: an updating. Biochemistry (Mosc). 2011;76(1):4-15.

Pavicic T, et al. Efficacy of cream-based novel formulations of hyaluronic acid of different molecular weights in anti-wrinkle treatment. J Drugs Dermatol. 2011;10(9):990-1000.

Philipp-Dormston WG. Botulinum toxin in dermatology. Hautarzt. 2014;65(2):133-45.

Plumb GW, et al. Are whole extracts and purified glucosinolates from cruciferous vegetables antioxidants? Free Radic Res. 1996;25:75-86.

Prahl S, et al. Aging skin is functionally anaerobic: importance of coenzyme Q10 for anti aging skin care. Biofactors. 2008;32(1-4):245-55.

R

Rhodes LE, et al. Dietary fish oil reduces basal and ultraviolet B-generated levels in skin and increases the threshold to provocation of polymorphic light eruption. J Invest Dermatol. 1995;105(4):532-535.

Riby JE, et al. The major cyclic trimeric product of indole-3-carbinol is a strong agonist of the estrogen receptor signaling pathway. Biochemistry. 2000;39(5):910-8.

Rizwan M, et al. Tomato paste rich in lycopene protects against cutaneous photodamage in humans invivo: a randomized controlled trial. Br J Dermatol. 2011;164(1):154-62.

Röck K, et al. Collagen fragments inhibit hyaluronan synthesis in skin fibroblasts in response to ultraviolet B (UVB): new insights into mechanisms of matrix remodeling. J Biol Chem. 2011;286(20):18268-76.

Rohdewald P. A review of the French maritime pine bark extract (Pycnogenol), a herbal medication with a diverse pharmacology. Int J Clin Pharmacol Ther. 2002;40(4):158-68.

Rozio, C. Nutrients in Oranges Help Protect Against Several Cancers for Up to 24 Hours After Eating. April 2005. http://www.sunkist.com/press/release-nutrients-in-oranges-help-protect-against-several-cancers-for-up-to-24-hours-after-eating_51.aspx

S

Saliou C et al. Solar ultraviolet-induced erythema in human skin and nuclear factor-kappa-B-dependent gene expression in keratinocytes are modulated by a French maritime pine bark extract. Free Rad Biol Med. 2001;30:154-160.

Schmidt JB, et al. Treatment of skin ageing symptoms in perimenopausal females with estrogen compounds. A pilot study. Maturitas. 1994;20(1):25-30.

Schmidt JB, et al. Treatment of skin aging with topical estrogens. Int J Dermatol. 1996;35(9):669-74.

Segger D et al. Supplementation with Evelle improves skin smoothness and elasticity in a double-blind, placebo-controlled study with 62 women. J Dermatol Treat. 2004;15(4):222-6.

Shah MG, et al. Estrogen and skin. An overview. Am J Clin Dermatol. 2001;2(3):143-50.

Smith RN, et al. The effect of a high-protein, low glycemic-load diet versus a conventional, high glycemic-load diet on biochemical parameters associated with acne vulgaris: a randomized, investigator-masked, controlled trial. J Am Acad Dermatol. 2007;57(2):247-56.

Solowiej E, et al. Chemoprevention of cancerogenesis—the role of sulforaphane. Acta Pol Pharm. 2003;60(1):97-100.

Stahl W, et al. Carotenoids and flavonoids contribute to nutritional protection against skin damage from sunlight. Mol Biotechnol. 2007;37(1):26-30.

Stanley M. Genital human papillomavirus infections: current and prospective therapies. J Gen Verol. 2012;93:681-91.

Suto A, et al. Alteration in proliferative and endocrine responsiveness of human mammary carcinoma cells by prototypic tumor-suppressing agents. Steroids. 1993;58(5):215-9.

T

Talalay P, et al. Chemoprotection against cancer by isothiocyanates and glucosinolates. Biochem Soc Trans. 1996;24:806-10.

Talalay P, et al. Sulforaphane mobilizes cellular defenses that protect skin against damage by UV radiation. Proc Natl Acad Sci. 2007;104(44):17500–17505.

Tausk F, et al. Stressed Mice Quicker To Get Skin Cancer. J Am Acad Dermatol. 2004;51(6):919-922.

Thangapazham RL, et al. Beneficial role of curcumin in skin diseases. Adv Exp Med Biol. 2007;595:343-57.

Tollesson A and A Frithz. Borage oil: An effective new treatment for infantile seborrhoiec dermatitis. Br J Dermatol. 1993;129:95.

Tollesson A and A Frithz. Transepidermal water loss and water content in the stratum corneum in infantile seborrhoeic dermatitis. Acta Derm Venereol. 1993;73:18.

U

Unlu NZ, et al. Carotenoid absorption from salad and salsa by humans is enhanced by the addition of avocado or avocado oil. J Nutr.2005;135(3):431-6.

V

Verhoeven DT, et al. A review of mechanisms underlying anticarcinogenicity by brassica vegetables. Chem Biol Interact. 1997;103:79-129. Review.

Verhoeven DT, et al. Epidemiological studies on brassica vegetables and cancer risk. Cancer Epidemiol Biomarkers Prev. 1996;5:733-48. Review.

Vitamin C cream improves redness from rosacea. Cosmetic Dermatol. 2001;14(2):35-38.

Y

Yasumuro M et al. Inhibition of melanogenesis by pine (Pinus pinaster) bark extract containing procyanidins. Manuscript in preparation. 2006.

Z

Zhang M, et al. Coenzyme Q(10) enhances dermal elastin expression, inhibits IL-1⊠ production and melanin synthesis in vitro. Int J Cosmet Sci. 2012;34(3):273-9.

Zhang Y, et al. A major inducer anticarcinogenic protective enzymes from broccoli: isolation and elucidation of structure. Proc Natl Acad Sci. 1992;89:2399-403.

Zhang Y, et al. High cellular accumulation of sulphoraphane, a dietary anticarcinogen, is followed by rapid transporter-mediated export as a glutathione conjugate. Biochem J. 2002;364:301-7.

Zhou JY, et al. An update on botulinum toxin a injections of trigger points for myofascial pain. Curr Pain Headache Rep. 2014;18(1):386.

Also by Lorna R. Vanderhaeghe

A Smart Woman's Guide to Hormones

A Smart Woman's Guide to Weight Loss

An A-Z Woman's Guide to Vibrant Health

A Smart Woman's Guide to Heart Health

Healthy Fats for Life:
Preventing and Treating Common Health
Problems with Essential Fatty Acids
with Karlene Karst, BSc, RD

Healthy Immunity:
Scientifically Proven Natural Treatments for
Conditions from A-Z

The Immune System Cure:
Nature's Way to Super-Powered Health
with Patrick JD Bouic, PhD

For more information about Lorna Vanderhaeghe, visit
www.hormonehelp.com

ACTIVE COLLAGEN™
Hydrolyzed Marine Collagen and Elastin Polypeptides

What to expect from this product:

- Reduces the depth of deep wrinkles
- Lifts and tones sagging areas
- Increases skin moisture
- Protects against free radical sun damage to skin
- Works fast with excellent clinical research
- Improves hair thickness
- Improves bone mineral density and joint disease
- Stops brittle nails
- Enhances collagen and elastin in 28 days

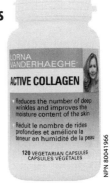

Over one-quarter of all the protein in the body is made up of collagen. Collagen is the protein that makes your bones, nails, teeth and hair strong. Collagen is also the main structural component of skin. Starting in our early 20s, however, collagen production declines by about one percent a year. Women in menopause are especially susceptible to collagen decline. Women lose as much as 30 percent of their skin collagen in the five years following menopause. And as if that is not bad enough, skin elasticity declines 0.55 percent per year after menopause. The effects of slowed collagen production are visibly obvious when skin loses its structure, sags and wrinkles.

A second yet equally important component of skin is called elastin. Elastin fibers form a matrix with collagen; together they allow the skin to flex and move. When we are young, the skin naturally renews its collagen and elastin. But with age, and as exposure to sun and environmental toxins damages the skin, this renewal rate slows down. Fortunately, it is possible to support collagen and elastic production.

Sourced from European waters to meet the highest standards of purity, Active Collagen is a marine ingredient composed of collagen and elastin polypeptides present in the same ratio that is naturally found in skin. Active Collagen has a synergistic anti-wrinkle action: when taken orally, collagen and elastin stimulate the skin to lift and tone sagging areas and minimize lines and wrinkles.

Active Collagen can also increase the moisture level of dry skin and fight aging related to free radical damage. Active Collagen polypeptides have a low molecular weight, making it water-soluble and easily absorbed by the body.

In a study of 43 women between the ages of 40 and 55 with crow's feet wrinkles, consumption of Active Collagen was found to decrease lines and wrinkles as well as to increase skin moisture. Two grams per day of either Active Collagen or placebo were ingested with a glass of water for 84 days. Subjects' forearm and face skin conditions were measured at day 0, day 28 and day 84. Day 28 through 84 were during winter months to simulate harsh winter conditions.

After 28 days, Active Collagen caused a significant decrease of 19 percent of the number of deep wrinkles in 71 percent of the subjects. Maximum benefit was achieved quickly. However, the placebo group experienced an increase in the number of deep wrinkles at both day 28 and day 84. Finally, Active Collagen caused a moisturizing effect on the skin. No side effects were reported. In conclusion, Active Collagen improved skin moisture and decreased the number of deep wrinkles. Active Collagen provided a protective effect against wrinkles compared to the placebo group (who actually experienced an increase in wrinkles).

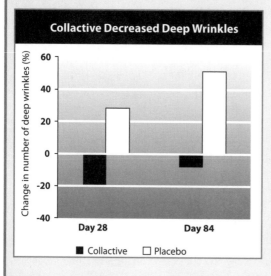

After 28 days, Active Collagen significantly decreased the number of wrinkles. At day 84, Active Collagen protected against wrinkles when exposed to harsh winter conditions.

FORMULA:

EACH CAPSULE CONTAINS:
Hydrolyzed marine collagen and elastin polypeptides (as Collactive™)
(Standardized to 85% collagen and 5% elastin) .... 500 mg

This product does not contain artificial preservatives, colors or sweeteners; no dairy, gluten, shellfish, soy, wheat or yeast. **GLUTEN FREE.**

SUGGESTED USAGE:

• Take 4 capsules per day with food.

CELADRIN™
Super Rich Skin Therapy Cream

What to expect from this product:

- Reduction of fine lines and wrinkles
- Treats psoriasis, eczema and rosacea
- Improves elasticity
- Moisturizes the skin
- Halts inflammation
- Contains hyaluronic acid and 10% Celadrin™

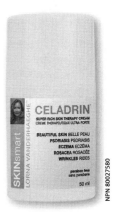

New research is proving that not only does CELADRIN™ perform in the treatment of arthritic conditions, sports injuries and other inflammatory disorders, but it also produces remarkable results in the fight against wrinkles, psoriasis, eczema, rosacea and other related inflammatory skin conditions.

CELADRIN™ and Wrinkles
It makes sense that this cream would have a positive effect on wrinkles due to its anti-inflammatory action. By calming the skin and halting inflammation (remember that inflammation promotes aging), we can reduce fine lines and wrinkles.

In a study of 28 subjects between the ages of 25 to 65, with an average age of 45, the cream was applied twice per day, morning and night. Each participant was evaluated after 21 days of application. The participants and the dermatologist noted measurable improvement including the reduction of wrinkles, and increase in skin permeability, and an improvement in the roughness and thickening of the skin, firmness and hydration.

CELADRIN™ Super Rich Skin Therapy Cream will reduce fine lines and wrinkles without reactions to fragrance additives; It is all natural, preservative and paraben-free. Hyaluronic acid is added for additional anti-wrinkle benefits.

CELADRIN™ and Psoriasis
Another double-blind, placebo-controlled study using CELADRIN™ cream for the treatment of psoriasis was performed over a 14 day period. Patients were asked to apply the cream to the affected area twice a day. Initial severity of skin scales, patchiness, redness, dryness, cracked and raised skin were recorded. Then after 7 and 14 days each patient visited the dermatologist who evaluated skin improvement. Each patient experienced a two level improvement based on the 6-point Liker scale (0 = no improvement, 5 = significant improvement).

This small pilot study found that those persons using CELADRIN™ cream experienced measurable improvement in their psoriasis.

Psoriasis is a difficult inflammatory skin condition to treat. CELADRIN™ Super Rich Skin Therapy Cream has shown positive results and may provide the answer for those suffering from this inflammatory condition.

CELADRIN™ Super Rich Skin Therapy Cream also helps those with eczema, rosacea and other skin conditions as it halts inflammation and heals the skin.

FORMULA:

Water, CELADRIN™ 10%, Aloe Barbadensis Leaf Gel, Stearic Acid, Glycerin, Olea Europaea (Olive) Oil Unsaponifiables, Cetyl Alcohol, Stearyl Alcohol, Anthemis Nobilis Flower (Roman Chamomile) extract, Butyrospermum Parkii (Shea Butter), Panthenol, Simmondsia Chinensis (Jojoba) Seed Oil, Vitis Vinifera (Grape seed) Oil, Sodium Hydroxymethylglycinate, Lactoperoxidase & Glucose Oxidase & Glucose, Tocopherol (Vitamin E), Hydroxyethyl Cellulose, Citric Acid, Sodium Hyaluronate, Anthemis Nobilis (Roman Chamomile) Flower Oil, Lavandula Angustifolia (Lavender) Oil, Pelargonium Graveolens (Geranium) Flower Oil, Santalum Album (Sandalwood) Oil.

SUGGESTED USAGE:

- Adults and children 2 years of age or older: Apply to the affected area morning and night and throughout the day as needed.

Rosacea Treatment!

Dear Lorna,

I have rosacea which causes red bumps and acne like lesions on my chin, nose and cheeks. I want to thank you for CELADRIN Super Rich Skin Therapy Cream because since using it I have not had a flare up of the rosacea. – TD, BC

Dear Lorna,

My daughter has terrible eczema and we started using CELADRIN Super Rich Skin Therapy Cream along with GLA Skin Oil and we can't believe how her skin has cleared up in the last 3 months. – SJ, QC

COLLAGEN PLUS
Silicic Acid and Biotin

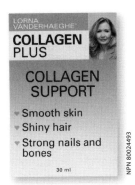

COLLAGEN PLUS

COLLAGEN SUPPORT

- Smooth skin
- Shiny hair
- Strong nails and bones

30 ml

NPN 80024493

What to expect from this product:

- Smooth, beautiful, glowing skin
- Thicker, stronger, healthier hair
- Strong nails and bones
- More flexible connective tissue
- Stops receding gums
- Use with BONE BOOSTER for osteoporosis
- Use with GLA SKIN OIL for skin

Why You Need Collagen
Over one-quarter of all the protein in the body is made up of collagen. Collagen is the protein that makes your bones, nails, teeth and hair strong. Collagen connective tissues run throughout the body and provide structure for your skeleton, tendons, cartilage and muscles, all of which support your internal organs and protect your softer tissues.

Collagen and Skin
Collagen also plays a critical role in skin health. You have probably noticed how baby skin is so soft and smooth. Youthful skin is abundant in collagen and elastin fibers that lock in moisture and keep the skin firm. As we age, however, collagen production naturally declines—by about 1 percent a year starting in our early 20s. Women in menopause are especially susceptible to collagen deficiency. Research shows that women lose as much as 30 percent of their skin collagen in the five years following menopause. And as if that is not bad enough, skin elasticity declines 0.55 percent per year after menopause. It is the loss of collagen that causes sagging skin and wrinkles.

Women spend billions of dollars on treatments such as skin fillers, laser and Botox. More so than any expensive treatment, however, it is possible to support beautiful skin and collagen production by choosing nutrients that provide the body with the necessary building blocks such as silicic acid and biotin.

The Silicon/Collagen Connection
Silicon is a trace mineral required by the body to make collagen. Specifically, silicon is converted into silicic acid that the body requires to manufacture collagen and elastin. Unfortunately, silicon from food, herbs and colloidal (gel) silica supplements is poorly absorbed, resulting in a lack of the building blocks required to make collagen. COLLAGEN PLUS contains silicic acid, which is directly used to make collagen. Within two to three months, you will notice an improvement in the smoothness of your skin and in the strength of your hair and nails.

COLLAGEN PLUS for Stronger Bones
Collagen is part of the matrix that ensures strong bones. One in four women has osteoporosis, and hip fractures are a leading cause of disability and sometimes

death. Smart women choose COLLAGEN PLUS as part of their healthy bone program. Receding gums are an early indicator of osteoporosis, and dentists have reported that COLLAGEN PLUS stops receding gums. Weak, fragile nails are also symptoms of poor bone health. To prevent osteoporosis, take COLLAGEN PLUS and MULTIsmart™. MULTIsmart™ contains all the bone-building nutrients, including the right forms of calcium, magnesium and vitamin D, along with all of your vitamins and minerals. If you have osteoporosis, take COLLAGEN PLUS, MULTIsmart™ and BONE BOOSTER.

BONE BOOSTER contains vitamin K2 MK-7 and vitamin D3 which are superior forms of nutrients to enhance bone health.

The "Plus" in COLLAGEN PLUS is Biotin

Like silicic acid, biotin is important for healthy hair, skin, nails and bones. Food sources of biotin include nuts, egg yolk, wheat bran, oat, barley, liver and brewer's yeast. However, the therapeutic amount of biotin required for healthy hair and nails exceeds that found in the typical diet. Topical biotin, often added to hair care products, is not as effective as biotin in capsule form. Supplemental biotin has been found to increase nail thickness and reduce splitting. COLLAGEN PLUS contains 50 micrograms of biotin in each drop.

FORMULA:

EACH DROP CONTAINS:
Silicon (silicic acid) .... 1 mg
Biotin... 50 mcg

This product does not contain irradiated rice flour, corn, dairy, soy, gluten, wheat, yeast, or artificial preservatives, colors or sweeteners. **VEGAN-FRIENDLY. GLUTEN-FREE.**

SUGGESTED USAGE:

- Mix 10 drops in a glass of juice or as directed by a health care practitioner. Take with food.

Incredible face lift!

Dear Lorna,

Yesterday I looked at myself in the mirror and noticed the fine lines on my forehead had softened quite noticeably. I did a double-take as I thought I was imagining this; went back and checked again a few times and they are definitely not as deep. I've had these lines since I was in my early twenties and no face cream or internal supplement has made this sort of improvement on my skin. I can only attribute this change to the fact that I've been taking Lorna's new COLLAGEN PLUS now for two weeks. I started the night of her visit to our Kamloops store after listening to the presentation. I have often marveled at how your skin glows Lorna and I think I know why now—it's the internal collagen supplementation. I hope that this will improve and soften the deeper smile lines I have around my mouth and eyes over time. I truly believe it has to be this product improving my skin as I haven't done any major diet changes. Thank you for your advice and great products! – KM, BC

GLA SKIN OIL™
Highly Concentrated GLA from Borage Oil

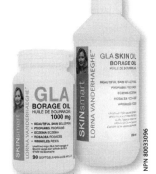

What to expect from this product:

- ♥ Ensures beautiful, smooth, glowing skin
- ♥ Improves calcium retention in bones
- ♥ Treats eczema, psoriasis and dermatitis
- ♥ Stops breast and period pain
- ♥ Stops cradle cap and dermatitis in infants
- ♥ Can also be applied topically along with oral treatment
- ♥ Now available in capsules too!

GLA is a Very Essential Fat

Essential fatty acids are good fats "essential" for optimal health. Unfortunately the North American diet is made up predominantly of bad fats from red meats and processed foods. To make matters worse when an enzyme in the body is impaired we can't make the good fats GLA, EPA or DHA. We can overcome this problem by eating fish or fish oils that contain EPA and DHA but when it comes to GLA the only way to get this important fatty acid is to take it in a nutritional supplement.

GLA (gamma linolenic acid) is found in borage oil (20 to 24%) and to a lesser extent evening primrose oil (8 to 10%). GLA is not found in food in high enough quantities to maintain our needs through diet alone.

GLA Eases Cramps and Breast Pain

GLA deficiency is a major cause of PMS. A healthy body creates GLA via an enzyme from fats such as sunflower oil into prostaglandins, which are hormone-like compounds that regulate blood clotting, inflammation and muscle contraction. Just before menstruation a cascade of prostaglandins are initiated in the uterus which causes the constriction of blood vessels and contractions that cause pain, cramps, nausea, vomiting, bloating and headaches that coincide with PMS. There are good prostaglandins and bad prostaglandins. Painful menstruation and breast pain are caused by low levels of good anti-inflammatory prostaglandins which are made from GLA. In many women with breast pain and terrible PMS their ability to make GLA is often impaired. One trial done at the breast clinic at the University of Hong Kong used GLA for the treatment of cyclical breast pain. Of the 66 women in the study 97% responded to treatment with GLA after 6 months. Further studies have found unusually low concentrations of GLA in the women suffering with period cramps and breast pain. The recommended dose is 1000 – 2000 mg of GLA per day.

GLA, Menopause and Skin

In women who have gone through menopause, the enzyme that converts food into GLA becomes impaired. GLA is a major component of beautiful skin. GLA makes your skin luminescent, dewy and glowing. The main reason our skin becomes dull and thick after menopause is due to the inability to make GLA. After menopause it is essential that we take a daily dose of GLA to ensure beautiful skin. As we age

GLA can reduce inflammation in the skin associated with wrinkled skin. Without sufficient GLA the skin becomes dry, rough and wrinkled. GLA is the beautiful skin oil.

GLA and Skin Health

GLA is a component of healthy skin. GLA helps to maintain the stability and fluidity of the natural water loss barrier in our skin. Skin disorders like eczema, psoriasis, rosacea, dermatitis, cradle cap, acne and dry skin occur. GLA is vital for keeping skin cells moist and strong improving the barrier function of the skin. In one study, 60 patients given 500 mg of GLA per day for eczema had a 90% improvement over 12 weeks. Eczema is a common problem in infants and children. GLA is safe for all ages without the side effects seen with steroid creams.

Cradle cap and infant dermatitis or dry crusts on the skin occur on the scalp, face, armpits, chest and groin area and can be treated with topical GLA oil. 48 infants with dermatitis were given twice daily applications of GLA oil for 6 weeks with complete relief. One teaspoon containing 500 mg of GLA should be applied twice a day.

GLA has also been found to inhibit male hormones in the skin that cause acne. GLA can be taken both internally and applied externally to acne prone areas with excellent results.

GLA and Breast Cancer

In a British study, women with advanced metastatic breast cancer taking Tamoxifen (a cancer drug that blocks estrogen) who also took GLA had a much faster response than those on Tamoxifen alone. Participants received 300 mg of GLA per day. The United Kingdom Cancer Research Campaign reports that GLA holds great potential in new cancer treatments.

GLA and Bone Density

Studies performed over 18 months found that when GLA was combined with calcium, GLA enhanced the absorption of calcium and improved bone density and prevented bone loss. Sixty five women with an average age of 79 years were given 600 mg of calcium glycinate/aspartate along with 1000 mg of GLA and had up to a 2% increase in bone density whereas the group receiving calcium alone lost 2 to 3% of bone over the 18 month period. Borage oil is the highest source of GLA. GLA SKIN OIL contains 500 mg of GLA per serving.

FORMULA:

EACH TEASPOON CONTAINS:
GLA (From organic Canadian borage seeds) .... 500 mg

SUGGESTED USAGE:

- Take 1 to 2 teaspoons daily with food and/or apply to the skin as needed.

Beautiful Skin from within!

Hi Lorna,

I noticed that since I went through menopause my skin is so dry and has wrinkled terribly. I heard you on the Fanny Kiefer show talking about GLA Skin Oil and I started taking 3 teaspoons a day and within 2 weeks my skin was glowing. My friends were asking what I had "done". Thank you!! All the best. – CK, ON